Welcome to Date Night Cookbook for Couples: Romantic Recipes to Rekindle Your Love with Delectable Dishes and Memorable Meals. This book is your culinary companion designed to transform your evenings into extraordinary dining experiences, where every meal becomes a celebration of love and connection. Whether you're newlyweds seeking to create a tradition of romantic dinners or long-time partners looking to reignite the spark, this cookbook is crafted to bring you closer together through the magic of food.

In today's fast-paced world, finding time to nurture your relationship can be challenging. However, sharing a meal has always been a profound way to bond and communicate. Cooking together allows you to collaborate, learn, and discover new flavors and techniques. It's a sensory experience that engages sight, smell, taste, and touch, making it the perfect activity for couples seeking to deepen their connection.

This cookbook is filled with a diverse array of recipes designed to suit every taste and occasion. From elegant appetizers that set the stage for a delightful evening to decadent desserts that add a sweet note to your night, each recipe is carefully curated to inspire romance and intimacy. You'll find simple, quick-to-prepare dishes for busy weeknights and more elaborate recipes for special occasions when you want to impress your partner.

But this book is more than just a collection of recipes. It's a guide to creating memorable dining experiences. Alongside each recipe, you'll find tips for setting the perfect ambiance, from choosing the right music and lighting to selecting wines that complement your meal. We also include conversation starters and fun activities to keep the evening lively and engaging.

Throughout this journey, we'll explore various cuisines and cooking styles, ensuring there's always something new and exciting to try. Whether you're in the mood for a cozy Italian dinner, a spicy Mexican feast, or a delicate Japanese-inspired meal, you'll find recipes that transport you and your partner to different parts of the world, all from the comfort of your kitchen.

In addition to rekindling your love, cooking together offers numerous benefits. It encourages teamwork, improves communication, and provides a sense of accomplishment. It's an opportunity to be creative, to experiment, and to share your successes (and occasional mishaps) with the person you love most.

So, light some candles, pour a glass of wine, and embark on a culinary adventure with the Date Night Cookbook for Couples. Let the recipes within these pages help you create not just meals, but memories. Here's to love, laughter, and many delicious date nights to come.

A Warm Welcome to Our Lovely Couples!

Congratulations on taking the first step towards making your evenings together even more special! We're thrilled to welcome you to the "Date Night Cookbook for Couples: Romantic Recipes to Rekindle Your Love with Delectable Dishes and Memorable Meals" .

This book is more than just a collection of recipes; it's an invitation to create unforgettable moments and deepen your bond through the joy of cooking and dining together. We hope that each dish you prepare will bring you closer, fill your hearts with warmth, and make every date night an occasion to remember.

Here's to love, laughter, and countless delicious adventures in the kitchen. Happy cooking and happy dating!

With love,
The Date Night Cookbook Team

What is the total cooking time, including prep time?

Prep Time : _______________

Cook Time : _______________

Servings : _______________

Ingredients:

- 2 lbs beef tenderloin, trimmed
- Salt and pepper
- 2 tbsp olive oil
- 8 oz mushrooms, finely chopped
- 1 shallot, minced
- 2 garlic cloves, minced
- 1 tbsp brandy or cognac
- 1 sheet frozen puff pastry, thawed
- 1 egg, beaten with 1 tbsp water

Is the recipe easy to follow?

1. Beef Wellington

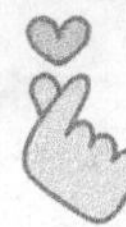

Procedure:

1. Season the beef tenderloin all over with salt and pepper.

2. Heat the olive oil in a skillet over high heat. Sear the beef on all sides until browned, about 2-3 minutes per side. Remove from heat and let cool completely.

3. In the same skillet, cook the mushrooms, shallot, and garlic over medium heat until the mushrooms have released their liquid and it has evaporated, about 5-7 minutes. Deglaze the pan with the brandy and cook for 1 more minute. Let cool completely.

4. On a lightly floured surface, roll out the puff pastry to a rectangle large enough to wrap around the beef. Spread the mushroom mixture in the center of the pastry. Place the beef tenderloin on top.

5. Wrap the pastry up and around the beef, pressing to seal the seam and edges. Place seam-side down. Brush the top and sides with the egg wash.

6. Bake at 400°F for 40-50 minutes, until the pastry is golden brown and the beef reaches your desired doneness (125°F for medium-rare).

7. Let rest 10 minutes before slicing and serving. Enjoy your romantic Beef Wellington dinner!

What is the total cooking time, including prep time?

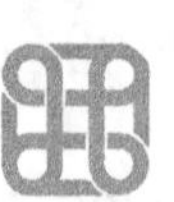 Prep Time : _______________

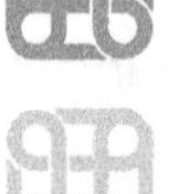 Cook Time : _______________

Servings : _______________

Ingredients:

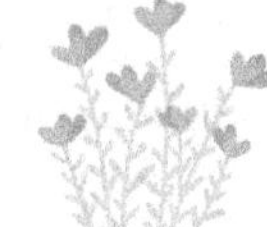

- 2 live lobsters (about 1-1.5 lbs each)
- 4 tbsp unsalted butter
- 1/4 cup finely chopped shallots
- 2 tbsp brandy or cognac
- 1/2 cup heavy cream
- 1/2 cup grated Gruyère cheese
- 2 egg yolks
- 2 tsp Dijon mustard
- Salt and pepper to taste
- Chopped parsley for garnish

Is the recipe easy to follow?

2. Lobster Thermidor

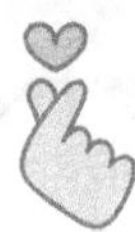

Procedure:

1. Bring a large pot of salted water to a boil. Add the live lobsters and cook for 8-10 minutes until bright red. Remove from water and let cool.

2. Crack the lobster shells and remove the meat from the tails and claws. Chop the meat into bite-sized pieces.

3. In a skillet, melt the butter over medium heat. Add the chopped shallots and cook for 2-3 minutes until softened.

4. Add the brandy and let it simmer for 1 minute. Then stir in the heavy cream and cook for 2-3 minutes until slightly thickened.

5. Remove the skillet from heat and stir in the Gruyère cheese, egg yolks, and Dijon mustard until well combined. Season with salt and pepper.

6. Gently fold in the chopped lobster meat until evenly coated.

7. Spoon the lobster Thermidor mixture back into the lobster shells. Place on a baking sheet.

8. Broil for 2-3 minutes until the tops are lightly browned.

9. Garnish with chopped parsley and serve immediately. Enjoy your romantic lobster dinner!

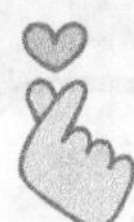

What are the critical points in the recipe (e.g., temperature control, timing)?

What is the total cooking time, including prep time?

Prep Time : _______________

Cook Time : _______________

Servings : _______________

Ingredients:

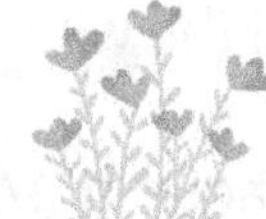

- 1 whole chicken, cut into 8 pieces (or 3 lbs chicken thighs and drumsticks)
- 4 slices bacon, diced
- 1 onion, diced
- 3 carrots, peeled and sliced
- 3 garlic cloves, minced
- 1 bottle red wine (Burgundy or Pinot Noir)
- 2 cups chicken stock
- 2 bay leaves
- 4 sprigs fresh thyme
- 1 lb mushrooms, quartered
- 2 tbsp butter
- 2 tbsp all-purpose flour
- Salt and pepper to taste
- Chopped parsley for garnish

Is the recipe easy to follow?

3. Coq au Vin

Procedure:

1. In a large Dutch oven or heavy bottomed pot, cook the bacon over medium heat until crispy. Remove bacon and set aside, reserving the bacon fat in the pot.

2. Season the chicken pieces all over with salt and pepper. Working in batches if needed, brown the chicken in the bacon fat on all sides, about 3-4 minutes per side. Remove chicken and set aside.

3. Add the onions, carrots and garlic to the pot. Cook for 5 minutes until softened.

4. Pour in the red wine and chicken stock. Add the bay leaves and thyme. Bring to a simmer.

5. Return the chicken pieces to the pot, cover and simmer for 45 minutes to 1 hour, until the chicken is very tender.

6. Remove the chicken from the pot and set aside. Discard the bay leaves and thyme sprigs.

7. In a small bowl, whisk together the butter and flour to make a paste. Slowly whisk this into the simmering sauce to thicken it.

8. Add the mushrooms and cooked bacon back to the pot. Simmer for 10 more minutes.

9. Return the chicken to the pot and heat through.

10. Serve the Coq au Vin over mashed potatoes or buttered egg noodles. Garnish with chopped parsley.

Enjoy this classic, comforting French dish for your romantic date night!

What are the critical points in the recipe (e.g., temperature control, timing)?

What is the total cooking time, including prep time?

Prep Time : _______________

Cook Time : _______________

Servings   : _______________

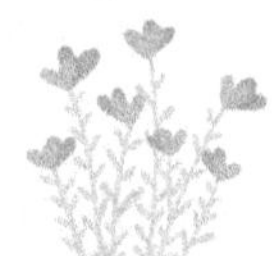

Ingredients:

Risotto:
- 4 cups chicken or vegetable broth
- 2 tbsp olive oil
- 1 onion, finely chopped
- 1 cup Arborio rice
- 1/2 cup dry white wine
- 1/2 cup grated Parmesan cheese
- 2 tbsp butter
- Salt and pepper to taste

Seared Scallops:
- 12 large sea scallops, patted dry
- 2 tbsp olive oil
- 2 tbsp butter
- Salt and pepper

Is the recipe easy to follow?

4. Seared scallops with risotto

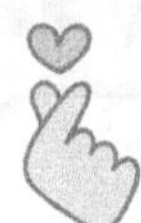

Procedure:

For the Risotto:
1. In a saucepan, bring the broth to a simmer and keep it warm over low heat.

2. In a large skillet, heat the olive oil over medium heat. Add the onion and cook for 3-4 minutes until translucent.

3. Add the Arborio rice and stir to coat with the oil. Cook for 2 minutes.

4. Pour in the white wine and stir constantly until the wine is absorbed, about 2 minutes.

5. Ladle in 1/2 cup of the warm broth and stir constantly until the liquid is absorbed. Continue this process, adding 1/2 cup of broth at a time, until the rice is tender and creamy, about 20-25 minutes total.

6. Remove from heat and stir in the Parmesan and butter until melted and combined. Season with salt and pepper.

For the Scallops:
1. Pat the scallops very dry with paper towels and season with salt and pepper.
2. Heat the olive oil and butter in a large skillet over high heat.
3. When the oil is shimmering, add the scallops in a single layer, making sure not to overcrowd the pan.
4. Sear the scallops for 2-3 minutes per side until golden brown.

To Serve:
Spoon the creamy risotto onto plates and top with the seared scallops. Garnish with extra Parmesan, chopped parsley, or lemon wedges if desired. Enjoy this elegant and romantic seafood and risotto dish!

What is the total cooking time, including prep time?

Prep Time : _______________

Cook Time : _______________

Servings   : _______________

Ingredients:

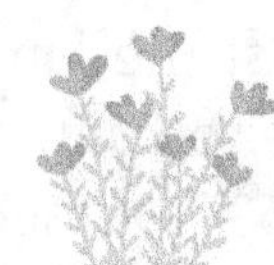

Truffle Butter:
- 1/2 cup unsalted butter, softened
- 2 tbsp finely chopped fresh parsley
- 1 tbsp finely chopped fresh thyme
- 1 tbsp finely chopped shallot
- 1 tsp truffle oil
- 1/4 tsp salt
- 1/4 tsp black pepper

Filet Mignon:
- 2 (6-8 oz) filet mignon steaks, about 1-inch thick
- 2 tbsp olive oil
- Salt and pepper to taste

Is the recipe easy to follow?

5. Filet mignon with truffle butter

Procedure:

For the Truffle Butter:

1. In a small bowl, combine the softened butter, parsley, thyme, shallot, truffle oil, salt and pepper. Mix well until fully incorporated.

2. Scoop the butter onto a piece of parchment paper or plastic wrap. Roll into a log shape and refrigerate until firm, at least 30 minutes.

For the Filet Mignon:

1. Pat the filet mignon steaks dry and season generously with salt and pepper on all sides.

2. Heat the olive oil in a large skillet or cast iron pan over high heat.

3. Sear the steaks for 2-3 minutes per side, until a nice brown crust forms.

4. Transfer the pan to a 400°F oven and roast for 8-12 minutes, flipping halfway, until the steaks reach your desired doneness (125°F for medium-rare).

5. Remove the steaks from the oven and let rest for 5-10 minutes.

6. Slice the chilled truffle butter into rounds and place on top of the warm filet mignon steaks. Allow the butter to melt slightly before serving.

To Serve:

Plate the filet mignon steaks with the melted truffle butter. Serve with roasted potatoes, asparagus, or a fresh salad for a complete romantic date night meal. Enjoy!

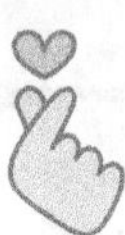

What are the critical points in the recipe (e.g., temperature control, timing)?

Procedure:

1. Preheat your oven to 400°F.

2. In a small bowl, mix together the olive oil, garlic, rosemary, and Dijon mustard. Season the lamb rack all over with salt and pepper.

3. Heat a large oven-safe skillet or cast iron pan over high heat. Sear the lamb rack on all sides until a nice brown crust forms, about 2-3 minutes per side.

4. Transfer the pan to the preheated oven. Roast the lamb for 15-20 minutes for medium-rare, or until it reaches your desired doneness (135°F for medium-rare, 140°F for medium).

5. Remove the lamb from the oven and let it rest for 10 minutes before slicing between the bones into individual chops.

6. Serve the rosemary lamb chops immediately, drizzling any pan juices over the top. Garnish with extra fresh rosemary if desired.

Pair this elegant rack of lamb with roasted potatoes, a fresh salad, and a nice glass of red wine for a truly romantic date night dinner. The rosemary and garlic flavors pair beautifully with the tender, juicy lamb. Enjoy!

What is the total cooking time, including prep time?

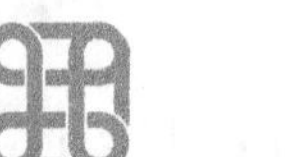

Prep Time : _______________

Cook Time : _______________

Servings   : _______________

Ingredients:

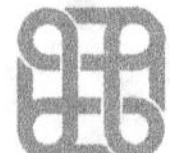
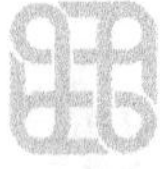
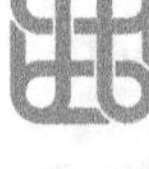
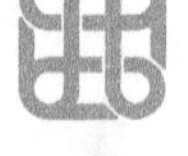

- 1 rack of lamb, frenched (8-9 ribs)
- 2 tbsp olive oil
- 3 garlic cloves, minced
- 2 tbsp fresh rosemary, finely chopped
- 1 tsp Dijon mustard
- Salt and pepper to taste

Is the recipe easy to follow?

6. Rack of lamb with rosemary

What is the total cooking time, including prep time?

Prep Time : _______________

Cook Time : _______________

Servings   : _______________

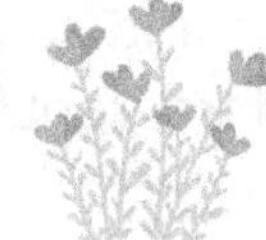

Ingredients:

- 12 oz jumbo pasta shells
- 15 oz ricotta cheese
- 10 oz frozen chopped spinach, thawed and squeezed dry
- 1 cup shredded mozzarella cheese, divided
- 1/2 cup grated Parmesan cheese
- 1 egg
- 2 garlic cloves, minced
- 1/4 tsp nutmeg
- Salt and pepper to taste
- 2 cups marinara sauce
- Fresh basil for garnish

Is the recipe easy to follow?

7. Spinach and ricotta stuffed shells

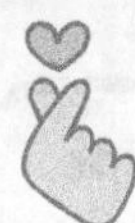

Procedure:

1. Preheat oven to 375°F. Cook the pasta shells according to package instructions until al dente. Drain and set aside.

2. In a large bowl, mix together the ricotta, spinach, 1/2 cup of the mozzarella, Parmesan, egg, garlic, nutmeg, salt and pepper until well combined.

3. Stuff each cooked pasta shell with a heaping tablespoon of the ricotta-spinach mixture.

4. Spread 1 cup of the marinara sauce in the bottom of a 9x13 baking dish. Arrange the stuffed shells in a single layer on top.

5. Pour the remaining 1 cup of marinara sauce over the top of the shells. Sprinkle with the remaining 1/2 cup of mozzarella cheese.

6. Bake for 25-30 minutes, until the cheese is melted and bubbly.

7. Let cool for 5 minutes, then serve the stuffed shells warm, garnished with fresh basil.

This comforting and cheesy stuffed shell dish is perfect for a romantic date night at home. Pair it with a fresh salad, garlic bread, and a nice glass of red wine for a complete Italian-inspired meal. Enjoy!

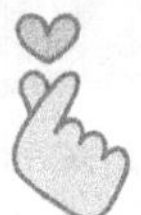

What are the critical points in the recipe (e.g., temperature control, timing)?

What is the total cooking time, including prep time?

Prep Time : _______________

Cook Time : _______________

Servings : _______________

Ingredients:

- 1 lb large shrimp, peeled and deveined
- 4 tbsp unsalted butter
- 3 tbsp olive oil
- 4 garlic cloves, minced
- 1/4 cup dry white wine
- 2 tbsp freshly squeezed lemon juice
- 2 tbsp chopped fresh parsley
- 1/4 tsp red pepper flakes (optional)
- Salt and pepper to taste
- Lemon wedges for serving

Is the recipe easy to follow?

8. Shrimp scampi

1. Pat the shrimp dry with paper towels and season with salt and pepper.

2. In a large skillet, melt 2 tbsp of the butter with the olive oil over medium-high heat.

3. Add the shrimp in a single layer and cook for 1-2 minutes per side, until just starting to turn pink. Transfer the shrimp to a plate.

4. Reduce the heat to medium and add the remaining 2 tbsp of butter to the skillet. Add the garlic and cook for 1 minute, stirring constantly, until fragrant.

5. Pour in the white wine and lemon juice. Bring to a simmer and cook for 2-3 minutes, scraping up any browned bits from the bottom of the pan.

6. Return the shrimp and any accumulated juices to the skillet. Cook for 2-3 minutes, tossing frequently, until the shrimp are cooked through.

7. Remove from heat and stir in the chopped parsley and red pepper flakes (if using). Taste and adjust seasoning with salt and pepper as needed.

8. Serve the shrimp scampi immediately, spooning the sauce over the top. Garnish with lemon wedges.

Serve this shrimp scampi over pasta, rice, or with crusty bread to soak up the delicious garlic-lemon sauce. It's an elegant and romantic date night dish that's sure to impress.

What is the total cooking time, including prep time?

Prep Time : ________________

Cook Time : ________________

Servings   : ________________

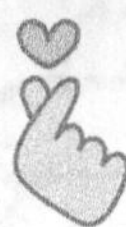

Ingredients:

- 1 (8 oz) round of brie cheese
- 2 tbsp honey
- 1/4 cup chopped walnuts or pecans
- 2 tbsp brown sugar
- 1 tsp ground cinnamon
- 1 baguette or crackers, for serving

Is the recipe easy to follow?

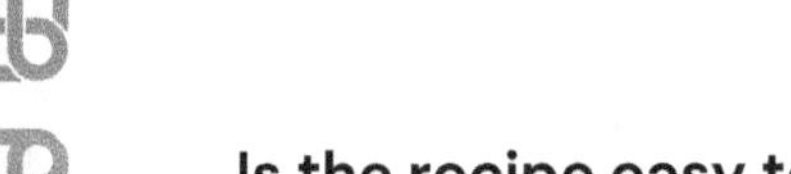
9. Baked brie with honey and nuts

Procedure:

1. Preheat your oven to 350°F. Line a baking sheet with parchment paper.

2. Place the round of brie cheese on the prepared baking sheet.

3. In a small bowl, mix together the honey, chopped nuts, brown sugar, and cinnamon until well combined.

4. Spoon the honey-nut mixture evenly over the top of the brie, allowing some to drip down the sides.

5. Bake for 12-15 minutes, until the brie is warm and softened.

6. Remove the baked brie from the oven and let it cool for 5 minutes.

7. Transfer the baked brie to a serving platter. Serve immediately with sliced baguette or crackers for dipping.

This warm, gooey baked brie is the perfect romantic appetizer for a date night. The sweet honey and crunchy nuts pair beautifully with the creamy, melted brie. It's an elegant and indulgent way to start your special evening. Enjoy!

What is the total cooking time, including prep time?

Prep Time   : ________________

Cook Time : ________________

Servings   : ________________

Ingredients:

- 18-24 fresh oysters, shucked, juices reserved
- 1/2 cup unsalted butter, softened
- 1/2 cup panko breadcrumbs
- 1/4 cup finely chopped parsley
- 2 tbsp finely chopped shallot
- 2 tbsp Pernod or other anise-flavored liqueur
- 2 garlic cloves, minced
- 1 tsp Worcestershire sauce
- 1/4 tsp cayenne pepper
- Salt and pepper to taste
- Lemon wedges for serving

Is the recipe easy to follow?

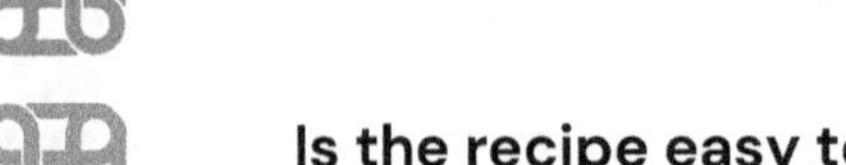

Procedure:

1. Preheat your oven to 450°F. Arrange the shucked oysters in their bottom shells on a baking sheet.

2. In a medium bowl, combine the softened butter, panko, parsley, shallot, Pernod, garlic, Worcestershire, cayenne, salt and pepper. Mix well until fully incorporated.

3. Spoon or pipe the flavored butter mixture evenly over the top of the oysters, covering them completely.

4. Bake for 8-10 minutes, until the topping is golden brown and the oysters are cooked through.

5. Carefully transfer the baked oysters Rockefeller to a serving platter. Drizzle any reserved oyster juices over the top.

6. Serve the oysters immediately, garnished with lemon wedges.

These decadent, creamy, and flavorful oysters Rockefeller make for an impressive and romantic appetizer for your date night. The combination of the briny oysters, rich butter, and aromatic herbs and spices is simply divine. Enjoy!

What is the total cooking time, including prep time?

Prep Time : _______________

Cook Time : _______________

Servings : _______________

Ingredients:

- 1 (2 lb) center-cut beef tenderloin, trimmed
- 2 tbsp olive oil
- 2 tsp coarse salt
- 1 tsp freshly ground black pepper
- 2 tbsp unsalted butter
- 2 garlic cloves, minced
- 2 sprigs fresh thyme
- 1/2 cup red wine
- 1 cup beef broth
- 2 tbsp Dijon mustard
- 2 tbsp heavy cream

Is the recipe easy to follow?

11. Châteaubriand for two

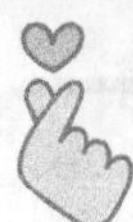

Procedure:

1. Preheat your oven to 400°F.

2. Pat the beef tenderloin dry and season all over with the salt and pepper.

3. Heat the olive oil in a large oven-safe skillet or cast iron pan over high heat. Sear the tenderloin on all sides until a nice brown crust forms, about 2-3 minutes per side.

4. Transfer the skillet to the preheated oven. Roast the Châteaubriand for 20-25 minutes, flipping halfway, until it reaches your desired doneness (125°F for medium-rare, 130°F for medium).

5. Remove the Châteaubriand from the oven and transfer it to a cutting board. Let it rest for 10-15 minutes.

6. In the same skillet, melt the butter over medium heat. Add the garlic and thyme and cook for 1 minute until fragrant.

7. Pour in the red wine and beef broth. Bring to a simmer and cook for 5-7 minutes, until the sauce has reduced by half.

8. Whisk in the Dijon mustard and heavy cream. Season with salt and pepper to taste.

9. Slice the Châteaubriand into thick, even slices. Serve the beef with the red wine sauce drizzled over the top.

This luxurious Châteaubriand dish is sure to impress your date. Serve it with roasted potatoes, sautéed greens, and a nice bottle of red wine for a truly romantic dinner.

What are the critical points in the recipe (e.g., temperature control, timing)?

What is the total cooking time, including prep time?

Prep Time : ___________________

Cook Time : ___________________

Servings : ___________________

- 4 large portobello mushroom caps, stems removed and chopped
- 2 tbsp olive oil
- 1 shallot, minced
- 2 garlic cloves, minced
- 1/2 cup breadcrumbs
- 1/2 cup grated Parmesan cheese
- 2 oz cream cheese, softened
- 2 tbsp chopped fresh basil
- Salt and pepper to taste
- Balsamic glaze for drizzling

Is the recipe easy to follow?

12. Stuffed portobello mushrooms

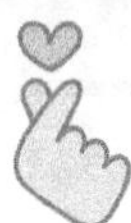

1. Preheat your oven to 400°F. Line a baking sheet with parchment paper.

2. Gently clean the portobello mushroom caps with a damp paper towel. Remove and chop the stems.

3. In a skillet, heat the olive oil over medium heat. Add the chopped mushroom stems, shallot, and garlic. Cook for 3-4 minutes until softened.

4. Remove the skillet from heat and stir in the breadcrumbs, Parmesan, cream cheese, and basil until well combined. Season with salt and pepper.

5. Arrange the portobello mushroom caps gill-side up on the prepared baking sheet. Spoon the filling mixture evenly into each mushroom cap.

6. Bake for 15-18 minutes, until the mushrooms are tender and the filling is hot and bubbly.

7. Remove the stuffed mushrooms from the oven and drizzle with balsamic glaze.

8. Serve the stuffed portobello mushrooms warm, garnished with extra basil if desired.

These savory, cheesy stuffed mushrooms make for a delightful vegetarian main or side dish for a romantic date night. The earthy portobellos pair beautifully with the creamy, herbed filling. Enjoy!

What are the critical points in the recipe (e.g., temperature control, timing)?

What is the total cooking time, including prep time?

Prep Time : _________________

Cook Time : _________________

Servings   : _________________

Ingredients:

- 3 lbs beef chuck, cut into 1-inch cubes
- 4 slices bacon, diced
- 1 onion, diced
- 3 carrots, peeled and sliced
- 3 garlic cloves, minced
- 2 cups red wine (such as Burgundy or Merlot)
- 2 cups beef broth
- 2 bay leaves
- 4 sprigs fresh thyme
- 1 lb mushrooms, quartered
- 2 tbsp butter
- 2 tbsp all-purpose flour
- Salt and pepper to taste
- Chopped parsley for garnish

Is the recipe easy to follow?

13. Beef bourguignon

Procedure:

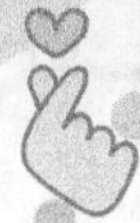

1. In a large Dutch oven or heavy bottomed pot, cook the bacon over medium heat until crispy. Remove the bacon and set aside, reserving the bacon fat in the pot.

2. Pat the beef cubes dry and season generously with salt and pepper. Working in batches if needed, sear the beef in the bacon fat until browned on all sides, about 3-4 minutes per batch. Transfer the seared beef to a plate.

3. Add the onions, carrots and garlic to the pot. Cook for 5 minutes until softened.

4. Pour in the red wine and beef broth. Add the bay leaves and thyme. Bring to a simmer.

5. Return the seared beef and any accumulated juices to the pot. Cover and transfer to a 325°F oven. Braise for 2-2.5 hours, until the beef is very tender.

6. In a small bowl, whisk together the butter and flour to make a paste. Slowly whisk this into the simmering sauce to thicken it.

7. Add the mushrooms and cooked bacon back to the pot. Simmer for 10 more minutes.

8. Taste and adjust seasoning with salt and pepper as needed.

9. Serve the beef bourguignon over mashed potatoes, egg noodles or crusty bread. Garnish with chopped parsley.

This rich, wine-braised beef dish is the perfect cozy and romantic meal for a date night. Pair it with a nice red wine for an authentic French experience.

What is the total cooking time, including prep time?

Prep Time : _______________

Cook Time : _______________

Servings   : _______________

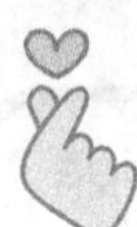

Ingredients:

- 1 lb salmon fillet, skin removed
- 1 sheet frozen puff pastry, thawed
- 4 oz cream cheese, softened
- 2 tbsp chopped fresh dill, plus more for garnish
- 1 egg, beaten with 1 tbsp water for egg wash
- Salt and pepper to taste

Is the recipe easy to follow?

14. Salmon en croûte

Procedure:

1. Preheat your oven to 400°F. Line a baking sheet with parchment paper.

2. Season the salmon fillet all over with salt and pepper.

3. In a small bowl, mix together the softened cream cheese and 2 tbsp of the chopped dill until well combined.

4. On a lightly floured surface, roll out the puff pastry sheet to a rectangle large enough to wrap around the salmon fillet.

5. Spread the cream cheese mixture evenly over the top of the salmon.

6. Place the salmon fillet, cream cheese side up, onto the center of the puff pastry. Fold the pastry up and over the salmon, pressing to seal the seams and edges.

7. Transfer the wrapped salmon en croûte to the prepared baking sheet, seam-side down. Brush the top and sides with the egg wash.

8. Bake for 25-30 minutes, until the pastry is golden brown and puffed.

9. Let the salmon en croûte rest for 5-10 minutes before slicing.

10. Slice and serve warm, garnished with additional fresh dill. Enjoy!

This elegant salmon dish wrapped in flaky puff pastry makes for a truly romantic and impressive date night dinner. Serve it with roasted vegetables, a fresh salad, and a glass of white wine for a complete meal.

What is the total cooking time, including prep time?

Prep Time : _______________

Cook Time : _______________

Servings   : _______________

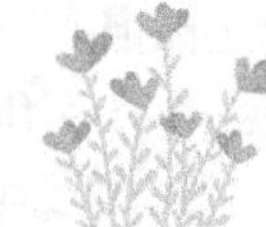

Ingredients:

- 4 boneless, skinless chicken breasts, pounded thin
- 1/2 cup all-purpose flour
- 4 tbsp unsalted butter, divided
- 3 tbsp olive oil
- 8 oz cremini or button mushrooms, sliced
- 1 shallot, minced
- 3 garlic cloves, minced
- 1 cup Marsala wine
- 1 cup chicken broth
- 2 tbsp heavy cream
- 2 tbsp chopped fresh parsley
- Salt and pepper to taste

Is the recipe easy to follow?

15. Chicken Marsala

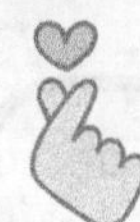

Procedure:

1. Season the pounded chicken breasts all over with salt and pepper. Dredge them in the flour, shaking off any excess.

2. In a large skillet, melt 2 tbsp of the butter with the olive oil over medium-high heat. Working in batches if needed, add the chicken and cook for 3-4 minutes per side until golden brown. Transfer the chicken to a plate.

3. Add the remaining 2 tbsp of butter to the skillet. Add the mushrooms and shallot, and cook for 3-4 minutes until the mushrooms are softened.

4. Stir in the garlic and cook for 1 minute until fragrant.

5. Pour in the Marsala wine and chicken broth. Bring to a simmer, scraping up any browned bits from the bottom of the pan.

6. Return the chicken and any accumulated juices to the skillet. Reduce heat to medium-low and simmer for 10-12 minutes, until the chicken is cooked through.

7. Remove the skillet from heat and stir in the heavy cream. Taste and adjust seasoning with salt and pepper as needed.

8. Serve the chicken Marsala immediately, garnished with the chopped parsley. Enjoy!

This rich and flavorful chicken Marsala is sure to impress your date. Serve it with roasted potatoes, buttered noodles, or a fresh salad for a complete romantic meal. The Marsala wine sauce is simply divine.

What are the critical points in the recipe (e.g., temperature control, timing)?

What is the total cooking time, including prep time?

Prep Time : ______________

Cook Time : ______________

Servings : ______________

Ingredients:

- 2 medium eggplants, sliced into 1/2-inch rounds
- Kosher salt
- 1 cup all-purpose flour
- 3 large eggs, beaten
- 2 cups panko breadcrumbs
- 1 cup grated Parmesan cheese, divided
- 2 tbsp olive oil, plus more for frying
- 3 cups marinara sauce
- 8 oz shredded mozzarella cheese

Is the recipe easy to follow?

16. Eggplant Parmesan

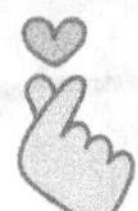

Procedure:

1. Preheat oven to 375°F. Grease a 9x13 baking dish.

2. Lay the eggplant slices in a single layer on paper towel-lined baking sheets. Sprinkle both sides generously with salt and let sit for 30 minutes to draw out moisture.

3. Set up a breading station with the flour, beaten eggs, and panko mixed with 1/2 cup of the Parmesan in 3 separate shallow dishes.

4. Working in batches, dredge the eggplant slices in the flour, dip in the egg, and then coat in the panko mixture, pressing to adhere.

5. In a large skillet, heat 1/4 inch of olive oil over medium-high heat. Fry the breaded eggplant slices in batches until golden brown on both sides, about 2-3 minutes per side. Transfer to a paper towel-lined plate.

6. Spread 1 cup of the marinara sauce in the bottom of the prepared baking dish. Arrange half of the fried eggplant slices in a single layer. Top with half of the remaining marinara sauce and half of the mozzarella and Parmesan cheeses.

7. Repeat the layers of eggplant, sauce, and cheeses.

8. Bake for 25-30 minutes, until the cheese is melted and bubbly.

9. Let the eggplant parmesan cool for 5-10 minutes before serving.

This comforting, cheesy eggplant parmesan is a delicious and romantic vegetarian option for your date night. Serve it with a fresh salad, garlic bread, and a nice glass of red wine for a complete Italian-inspired meal.

What is the total cooking time, including prep time?

Prep Time : _________________

Cook Time : _________________

Servings : _________________

Ingredients:

- 2 (8 oz) beef tenderloin steaks, about 1-inch thick
- 2 tbsp whole black peppercorns, crushed
- 2 tbsp olive oil
- 2 tbsp unsalted butter
- 1/2 cup brandy or cognac
- 1 cup beef broth
- 1/4 cup heavy cream
- Salt to taste

Is the recipe easy to follow?

17. Steak au poivre

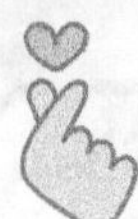

Procedure:

1. Pat the steaks dry and generously coat both sides with the crushed black peppercorns, pressing them in to adhere.

2. Heat the olive oil in a large skillet over high heat. When the oil is shimmering, add the steaks and sear for 2-3 minutes per side, until a nice crust forms.

3. Transfer the seared steaks to a plate and set aside.

4. Reduce the heat to medium and add the butter to the skillet. Once melted, carefully pour in the brandy or cognac. Allow it to simmer for 1-2 minutes.

5. Slowly whisk in the beef broth and heavy cream. Bring the sauce to a simmer and let it reduce for 5-7 minutes, until thickened slightly.

6. Return the seared steaks and any accumulated juices to the skillet. Spoon the sauce over the steaks.

7. Cook the steaks for an additional 2-4 minutes per side, flipping occasionally, until they reach your desired doneness (125°F for medium-rare, 130°F for medium).

8. Transfer the steaks to a cutting board and let rest for 5 minutes.

9. Slice the steaks and serve immediately, drizzled with the peppery brandy cream sauce. Season with salt to taste.

This classic steak au poivre is an elegant and romantic dish that's sure to impress your date. Serve it with roasted potatoes, sautéed greens, and a glass of red wine for a complete French-inspired meal.

Procedure:

What is the total cooking time, including prep time?

Prep Time : _______________

Cook Time : _______________

Servings   : _______________

Ingredients:

- 6 cups low-sodium chicken or vegetable broth
- 2 tbsp olive oil
- 1 lb mixed mushrooms (such as cremini, shiitake, oyster), sliced
- 1 shallot, minced
- 2 garlic cloves, minced
- 1 1/2 cups Arborio rice
- 1/2 cup dry white wine
- 1/2 cup grated Parmesan cheese, plus more for serving
- 2 tbsp unsalted butter
- 2 tbsp chopped fresh parsley
- Salt and pepper to taste

1. In a saucepan, bring the broth to a simmer over medium heat. Reduce heat to low to keep the broth warm.

2. In a large skillet, heat the olive oil over medium-high heat. Add the mushrooms and cook for 5-7 minutes, until browned and tender. Transfer the mushrooms to a plate.

3. Reduce the heat to medium and add the shallot and garlic to the skillet. Cook for 2-3 minutes until fragrant.

4. Add the Arborio rice and stir to coat with the oil. Cook for 2 minutes.

5. Pour in the white wine and cook, stirring constantly, until the wine is absorbed, about 2 minutes.

6. Ladle in 1/2 cup of the warm broth and stir constantly until the liquid is absorbed. Continue this process, adding 1/2 cup of broth at a time, until the rice is tender and creamy, about 20-25 minutes total.

7. Remove from heat and stir in the cooked mushrooms, Parmesan, butter, and parsley. Season with salt and pepper to taste.

8. Serve the mushroom risotto immediately, garnished with additional Parmesan if desired.

This rich and creamy mushroom risotto is an elegant and romantic date night dish. Pair it with a crisp white wine and a simple salad for a complete meal. The earthy mushrooms and indulgent Parmesan make this risotto truly special.

Is the recipe easy to follow?

18. Mushroom risotto

What is the total cooking time, including prep time?

Prep Time : _______________

Cook Time : _______________

Servings   : _______________

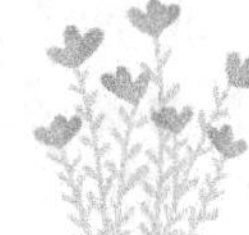

Ingredients:

- 4 (6 oz) flounder fillets
- 8 oz lump crabmeat, picked over for shells
- 1/2 cup panko breadcrumbs
- 1/4 cup grated Parmesan cheese
- 2 tbsp chopped fresh parsley
- 2 tbsp melted butter
- 1 tbsp lemon juice
- 1 garlic clove, minced
- Salt and pepper to taste
- Lemon wedges for serving

Is the recipe easy to follow?

19. Crab-stuffed flounder

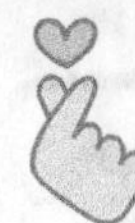

Procedure:

1. Preheat your oven to 400°F. Grease a baking dish or line with parchment paper.

2. In a medium bowl, gently mix together the crabmeat, panko, Parmesan, parsley, melted butter, lemon juice, and garlic. Season with salt and pepper.

3. Lay the flounder fillets flat in the prepared baking dish. Divide the crab stuffing evenly among the fillets, spooning it down the center.

4. Bake for 15-18 minutes, until the flounder is opaque and flakes easily with a fork, and the stuffing is hot and lightly browned on top.

5. Carefully transfer the crab-stuffed flounder to plates. Serve immediately, garnished with lemon wedges.

This elegant crab-stuffed flounder makes for a truly romantic and impressive date night dinner. The delicate white fish pairs beautifully with the rich, savory crab filling. Serve it with a fresh salad, roasted vegetables, and a crisp white wine for a complete meal.

The combination of the tender, flaky flounder and the decadent crab stuffing is sure to impress your date. Enjoy this special seafood dish together!

What is the total cooking time, including prep time?

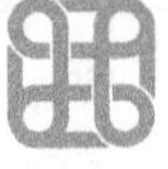
Prep Time : _________________

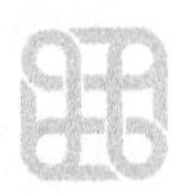
Cook Time : _________________

Servings   : _________________

Ingredients:

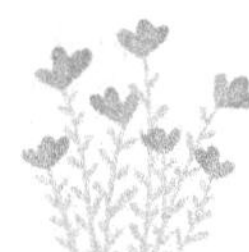

Duck:
- 2 (8 oz) duck breasts, skin on
- Salt and pepper

Cherry Sauce:
- 1 cup fresh or frozen pitted cherries
- 1/2 cup red wine
- 2 tbsp balsamic vinegar
- 2 tbsp honey
- 1 tbsp unsalted butter
- 1 garlic clove, minced
- Salt and pepper to taste

Is the recipe easy to follow?

20. Roasted duck breast with cherry sauce

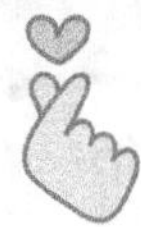

Procedure:

For the Duck:
1. Pat the duck breasts dry and score the skin in a crosshatch pattern, being careful not to cut into the meat. Season generously with salt and pepper.

2. Place the duck breasts skin-side down in a cold cast iron or oven-safe skillet. Turn the heat to medium and cook for 12-15 minutes, rendering the fat and crisping the skin.

3. Flip the duck breasts and transfer the skillet to a 400°F oven. Roast for 8-10 minutes for medium-rare, or until the duck reaches your desired doneness.

4. Remove the duck from the oven and let rest for 5-10 minutes before slicing.

For the Cherry Sauce:
1. In a small saucepan, combine the cherries, red wine, balsamic vinegar, and honey. Bring to a simmer over medium heat.

2. Cook for 10-12 minutes, stirring occasionally, until the sauce has thickened slightly.

3. Remove from heat and stir in the butter and garlic. Season with salt and pepper to taste.

To Serve:
Slice the roasted duck breasts and arrange on plates. Drizzle the warm cherry sauce over the top. Serve immediately.

This elegant dish of crispy-skinned duck breast paired with a sweet and tangy cherry sauce is sure to impress your date. Serve it with roasted potatoes, sautéed greens, and a glass of red wine for a truly romantic dinner.

What are the critical points in the recipe (e.g., temperature control, timing)?

What is the total cooking time, including prep time?

Prep Time : ________________

Cook Time : ________________

Servings : ________________

Ingredients:

- 1 lb mixed mushrooms (such as cremini, shiitake, oyster), finely chopped
- 1 onion, finely chopped
- 3 garlic cloves, minced
- 1 tbsp olive oil
- 1 tsp dried thyme
- Salt and pepper to taste
- 1 sheet frozen puff pastry, thawed
- 1 lb mixed roasted vegetables (such as sweet potato, zucchini, bell pepper), chopped
- 1 egg, beaten with 1 tbsp water for egg wash

Is the recipe easy to follow?

21. Vegetable Wellington

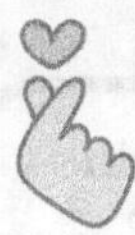

Procedure:

1. Preheat your oven to 400°F. Line a baking sheet with parchment paper.

2. In a large skillet, heat the olive oil over medium heat. Add the chopped mushrooms, onion, and garlic. Cook for 8-10 minutes, stirring occasionally, until the mushrooms have released their liquid and the onions are translucent.

3. Season the mushroom mixture with the thyme, salt, and pepper. Remove from heat and let cool slightly.

4. On a lightly floured surface, roll out the puff pastry sheet to a rectangle large enough to wrap around the vegetable filling.

5. Spread the cooled mushroom mixture evenly in the center of the pastry. Top with the chopped roasted vegetables.

6. Fold the pastry up and over the vegetable filling, pressing to seal the seams and edges. Place the wrapped Wellington seam-side down on the prepared baking sheet.

7. Brush the top and sides of the Wellington with the egg wash.

8. Bake for 30-35 minutes, until the pastry is golden brown and puffed.

9. Let the Vegetable Wellington rest for 5-10 minutes before slicing and serving.

This elegant vegetable Wellington makes for a delicious and impressive meat-free main course for a romantic date night. Serve it with a fresh salad, roasted potatoes, and a glass of white wine for a complete meal.

What is the total cooking time, including prep time?

Prep Time : ________________

Cook Time : ________________

Servings   : ________________

Ingredients:

- 4 veal shanks (about 3 lbs total)
- Salt and pepper
- 2 tbsp olive oil
- 1 onion, diced
- 2 carrots, peeled and diced
- 2 celery stalks, diced
- 4 garlic cloves, minced
- 1 cup dry white wine
- 1 (28 oz) can crushed tomatoes
- 2 cups beef or chicken broth
- 2 bay leaves
- 2 sprigs fresh thyme
- Gremolata (chopped parsley, lemon zest, garlic) for serving

Is the recipe easy to follow?

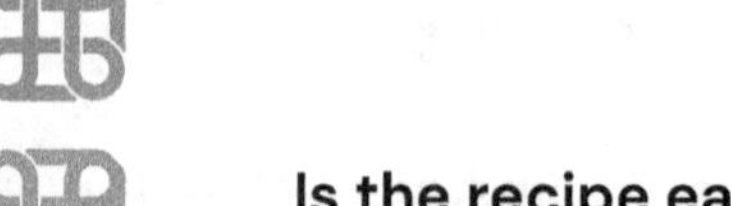

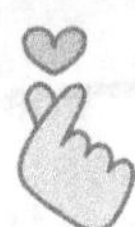

Procedure:

1. Pat the veal shanks dry and season generously with salt and pepper.

2. Heat the olive oil in a large Dutch oven or heavy bottomed pot over medium-high heat. Working in batches if needed, sear the veal shanks on all sides until browned, about 3-4 minutes per side. Transfer to a plate.

3. Reduce heat to medium and add the onion, carrots, celery and garlic to the pot. Cook for 5-7 minutes until softened.

4. Pour in the white wine and use a wooden spoon to scrape up any browned bits from the bottom of the pot. Let the wine simmer for 2-3 minutes.

5. Add the crushed tomatoes, broth, bay leaves and thyme. Return the seared veal shanks to the pot and bring to a simmer.

6. Cover the pot, transfer to a 325°F oven and braise for 2-2.5 hours, until the meat is very tender and falling off the bone.

7. Remove the pot from the oven. Transfer the veal shanks to a serving platter.

8. Discard the bay leaves and thyme sprigs. Taste the sauce and adjust seasoning with salt and pepper as needed.

9. Serve the osso buco warm, spooning the sauce over the top. Garnish with the gremolata.

This classic Italian osso buco is a wonderfully rich and flavorful dish, perfect for an elegant and romantic date night. Serve it over creamy polenta or buttered egg noodles for a complete meal.

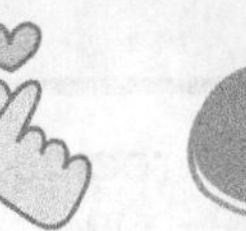

What are the critical points in the recipe (e.g., temperature control, timing)?

What is the total cooking time, including prep time?

Prep Time : ___________________

Cook Time : ___________________

Servings : ___________________

Ingredients:

Butternut Squash Ravioli

For the Ravioli Filling:
- 1 small butternut squash, peeled, seeded and cubed (about 2 cups)
- 2 tbsp unsalted butter
- 2 tbsp grated Parmesan cheese
- 1 tsp chopped fresh sage
- 1/4 tsp ground nutmeg
- Salt and pepper to taste

For the Pasta Dough:
- 2 cups all-purpose flour
- 3 large eggs
- 1 tsp olive oil
- 1/2 tsp salt

For Serving:
- 4 tbsp unsalted butter
- 1/4 cup toasted pine nuts
- Grated Parmesan cheese
- Chopped fresh sage

23. Butternut squash ravioli

Make the Ravioli Filling:
1. Steam or roast the butternut squash until very soft. Mash or puree until smooth.
2. In a bowl, mix the mashed squash with the butter, Parmesan, sage, nutmeg, salt and pepper until well combined.

Make the Pasta Dough:
1. On a clean surface, make a well with the flour. Crack the eggs into the well and add the olive oil and salt.
2. Using a fork, gradually incorporate the flour into the egg mixture until a shaggy dough forms.
3. Knead the dough for 5-7 minutes until smooth and elastic. Cover and let rest for 30 minutes.

Assemble the Ravioli:
1. Divide the dough into 4 pieces. Working with one piece at a time (keep the rest covered), roll the dough very thin using a pasta machine or rolling pin.
2. Place tablespoon-sized dollops of the butternut squash filling evenly across the dough, leaving space between each.
3. Brush the dough around the filling with water. Fold the dough over to cover the filling and press firmly to seal.
4. Use a ravioli cutter or knife to cut out the individual ravioli. Place on a lightly floured baking sheet.

Cook the Ravioli:
1. Bring a large pot of salted water to a boil. Gently add the ravioli and cook for 2-3 minutes until they float to the top.
2. In a skillet, melt the butter over medium heat. Add the cooked ravioli and toss to coat.
3. Serve the butternut squash ravioli warm, topped with toasted pine nuts, Parmesan, and chopped sage.

What is the total cooking time, including prep time?

Prep Time : _______________

Cook Time : _______________

Servings   : _______________

Ingredients:

- 1 lb mussels, scrubbed and debearded
- 1 lb large shrimp, peeled and deveined
- 1 lb calamari, bodies sliced into rings, tentacles left whole
- 1 tbsp olive oil
- 1 onion, diced
- 3 garlic cloves, minced
- 1 tsp smoked paprika
- 1/2 tsp saffron threads
- 1 cup short-grain Spanish rice (such as Bomba or Calasparra)
- 2 cups warm chicken or seafood broth
- 1 (14 oz) can diced tomatoes
- 1 cup frozen peas
- 1 lemon, cut into wedges for serving
- Chopped parsley for garnish

Is the recipe easy to follow?

24. Seafood paella

Procedure:

1. In a large paella pan or skillet, bring 1 cup of water to a boil. Add the mussels, cover and cook for 2-3 minutes until they start to open. Discard any that don't open. Remove the mussels from the pan and set aside.

2. In the same pan, heat the olive oil over medium-high heat. Add the onion and cook for 3-4 minutes until translucent.

3. Stir in the garlic, paprika and saffron. Cook for 1 minute until fragrant.

4. Add the rice and stir to coat with the oil. Pour in the broth and diced tomatoes. Bring to a simmer.

5. Reduce heat to medium-low, cover and cook for 15 minutes, until the rice is almost tender.

6. Nestle the shrimp, calamari and reserved mussels into the rice. Cover and cook for 5-7 minutes more, until the seafood is cooked through.

7. Remove from heat and stir in the frozen peas. Let stand, covered, for 5 minutes.

8. Serve the seafood paella immediately, garnished with chopped parsley and lemon wedges.

This vibrant and flavorful seafood paella is a showstopping dish perfect for a romantic date night. Serve it with a crisp white wine and some crusty bread for soaking up the delicious broth. Enjoy!

What is the total cooking time, including prep time?

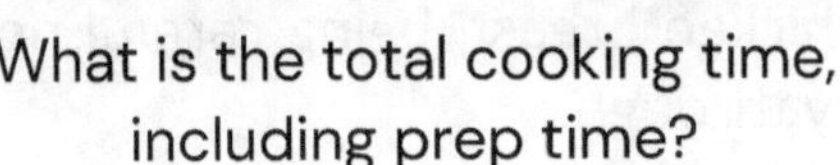

Prep Time   : _______________

Cook Time : _______________

Servings   : _______________

Ingredients:

- 2 lbs beef tenderloin, trimmed
- 2 tbsp olive oil
- Salt and pepper
- 1 shallot, minced
- 2 garlic cloves, minced
- 1 cup dry red wine
- 1 cup beef broth
- 2 tbsp unsalted butter
- 2 tbsp chopped fresh parsley

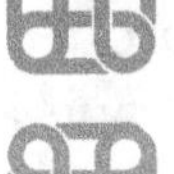
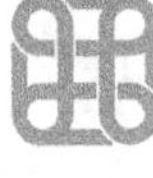

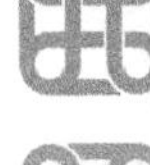
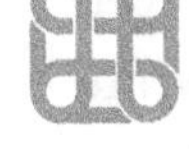

Is the recipe easy to follow?

25. *Beef tenderloin with red wine sauce*

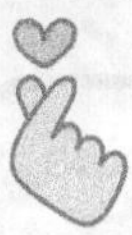

Procedure:

1. Preheat your oven to 400°F.

2. Pat the beef tenderloin dry and season generously all over with salt and pepper.

3. Heat the olive oil in a large oven-safe skillet or cast iron pan over high heat. Sear the tenderloin on all sides until a nice brown crust forms, about 2-3 minutes per side.

4. Transfer the skillet to the preheated oven. Roast the tenderloin for 20-25 minutes, flipping halfway, until it reaches your desired doneness (125°F for medium-rare, 130°F for medium).

5. Remove the tenderloin from the oven and transfer it to a cutting board. Let it rest for 10-15 minutes.

6. Meanwhile, return the skillet to medium heat on the stovetop. Add the shallot and garlic and cook for 1 minute until fragrant.

7. Pour in the red wine and beef broth. Bring to a simmer and cook for 5-7 minutes, until the sauce has reduced by half.

8. Remove the skillet from heat and whisk in the butter until melted and incorporated. Season the sauce with salt and pepper to taste.

9. Slice the beef tenderloin into thick, even slices. Arrange on a serving platter and drizzle the red wine sauce over the top.

10. Garnish with the chopped fresh parsley.

Serve this elegant beef tenderloin with roasted potatoes, sautéed greens, and a nice bottle of red wine for a truly romantic date night dinner. The rich, velvety red wine sauce is the perfect complement to the tender, juicy beef.

What is the total cooking time, including prep time?

Prep Time : ________________

Cook Time : ________________

Servings   : ________________

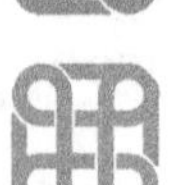
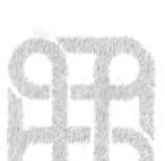
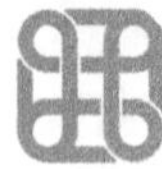
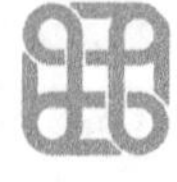

Ingredients:

- 4 boneless, skinless chicken breasts
- 4 oz crumbled feta cheese
- 1 cup fresh spinach, chopped
- 2 tbsp cream cheese, softened
- 2 garlic cloves, minced
- 1 tsp dried oregano
- Salt and pepper to taste
- 2 tbsp olive oil
- 1/4 cup white wine or chicken broth

Is the recipe easy to follow?

26. Stuffed chicken breast with spinach and feta

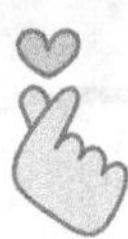

Procedure:

1. Preheat your oven to 400°F. Grease a baking dish or line with parchment paper.

2. Use a sharp knife to cut a pocket into the side of each chicken breast, being careful not to cut all the way through.

3. In a bowl, mix together the feta, spinach, cream cheese, garlic, and oregano. Season with salt and pepper.

4. Stuff each chicken breast pocket evenly with the spinach-feta mixture.

5. Heat the olive oil in a large oven-safe skillet over medium-high heat. Sear the stuffed chicken breasts for 2-3 minutes per side until golden brown.

6. Transfer the skillet to the preheated oven. Bake for 20-25 minutes, until the chicken is cooked through and the filling is hot.

7. Remove the chicken from the oven and transfer to a serving platter.

8. Place the skillet back on the stovetop over medium heat. Pour in the white wine or broth and use a wooden spoon to scrape up any browned bits from the bottom of the pan. Let the sauce simmer for 2-3 minutes.

9. Spoon the pan sauce over the stuffed chicken breasts before serving.

This elegant stuffed chicken dish is sure to impress your date. Serve it with roasted potatoes, a fresh salad, and a glass of white wine for a complete romantic meal. The creamy spinach and feta filling is the perfect complement to the juicy chicken.

What is the total cooking time, including prep time?

Prep Time : _______________

Cook Time : _______________

Servings   : _______________

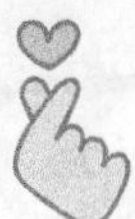

Ingredients:

- 4 (6-8 oz) lobster tails, thawed if frozen
- 4 tbsp unsalted butter, melted
- 2 tbsp lemon juice
- 2 garlic cloves, minced
- 1 tsp paprika
- 1/4 tsp cayenne pepper (optional)
- Salt and pepper to taste
- Lemon wedges for serving

Is the recipe easy to follow?

27. Grilled lobster tails

Procedure:

1. Preheat your grill to medium-high heat.

2. Using kitchen shears, cut along the center of the top of each lobster tail shell, being careful not to cut all the way through.

3. Gently pull the shell apart to expose the lobster meat, leaving the meat attached at the base.

4. In a small bowl, whisk together the melted butter, lemon juice, garlic, paprika, and cayenne (if using). Season with salt and pepper.

5. Brush the lobster meat generously with the garlic-butter mixture.

6. Grill the lobster tails meat-side up for 8-10 minutes, basting with more of the garlic-butter halfway through, until the meat is opaque and cooked through.

7. Transfer the grilled lobster tails to a serving platter. Serve immediately with lemon wedges on the side.

Provide any additional tips:
- Be careful not to overcook the lobster, as it can become tough and rubbery. Keep a close eye on it while grilling.
- For an extra decadent touch, you can top the grilled lobster with a pat of compound butter before serving.
- Serve the grilled lobster tails with a side of roasted asparagus or a fresh salad for a complete romantic meal.

This simple yet elegant grilled lobster tails dish is sure to impress your date. The sweet, tender lobster meat paired with the garlic-butter sauce makes for a truly indulgent and romantic seafood dinner.

What are the critical points in the recipe (e.g., temperature control, timing)?

What is the total cooking time, including prep time?

Prep Time : ___________________

Cook Time : ___________________

Servings   : ___________________

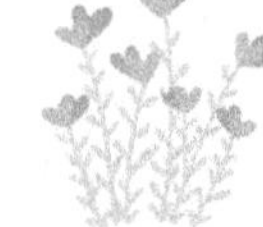

Ingredients:

- 9 lasagna noodles
- 1 tbsp olive oil
- 1 onion, diced
- 3 cloves garlic, minced
- 8 oz mushrooms, sliced
- 1 red bell pepper, diced
- 1 zucchini, diced
- 1 15oz can diced tomatoes
- 1 6oz can tomato paste
- 1 tsp dried basil
- 1 tsp dried oregano
- Salt and pepper to taste
- 15 oz ricotta cheese
- 1 egg
- 1/4 cup grated Parmesan cheese
- 2 cups shredded mozzarella cheese

Is the recipe easy to follow?

28. Vegetarian lasagna

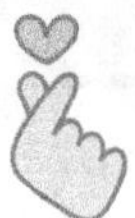

Procedure:

1. Preheat oven to 375°F. Cook the lasagna noodles according to package instructions. Drain and set aside.

2. In a large skillet, heat the olive oil over medium heat. Add the onion and garlic and sauté for 2-3 minutes until fragrant.

3. Add the mushrooms, bell pepper, and zucchini. Sauté for 5-7 minutes until vegetables are tender.

4. Stir in the diced tomatoes, tomato paste, basil, oregano, salt and pepper. Simmer for 10 minutes.

5. In a medium bowl, mix together the ricotta cheese, egg, and Parmesan.

6. Spread 1 cup of the vegetable sauce in the bottom of a 9x13 baking dish. Layer 3 lasagna noodles on top. Spread half of the ricotta mixture over the noodles, then top with 1 cup of the vegetable sauce and 1/2 cup mozzarella.

7. Repeat the noodle, ricotta, sauce, and mozzarella layers. Top with the remaining 3 noodles and the rest of the vegetable sauce.

8. Cover with foil and bake for 30 minutes. Remove foil and bake for 15 more minutes until hot and bubbly.

9. Let stand for 10 minutes before serving. Garnish with fresh basil if desired.

Enjoy this delicious and romantic vegetarian lasagna with your date! The layers of vegetables, creamy ricotta, and melted cheese make it a comforting and indulgent meal.

What is the total cooking time, including prep time?

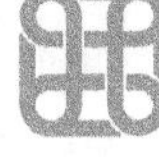
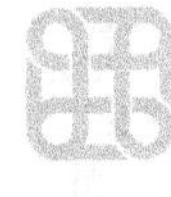
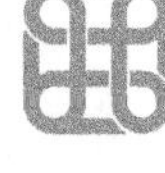
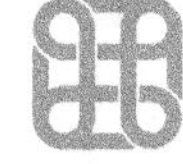

Prep Time : _________________

Cook Time : _________________

Servings   : _________________

Ingredients:

- 2 duck breasts, skin-on
- Salt and pepper
- 2 tbsp olive oil
- 1 shallot, minced
- 1 cup fresh or frozen blackberries
- 1/4 cup balsamic vinegar
- 2 tbsp honey
- 1 tbsp Dijon mustard
- 2 tbsp butter
- Fresh thyme for garnish

Is the recipe easy to follow?

29. Pan-seared duck with blackberry sauce

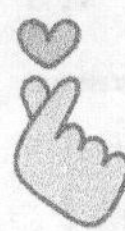

Procedure:

1. Pat the duck breasts dry and season generously with salt and pepper on both sides.

2. Heat the olive oil in a large skillet over medium-high heat. When the oil is hot, add the duck breasts skin-side down. Cook for 5-7 minutes until the skin is crispy and golden brown.

3. Flip the duck breasts and cook for another 3-5 minutes for medium-rare doneness. Transfer the duck to a cutting board and let rest for 5 minutes.

4. Reduce the heat to medium and add the shallot to the skillet. Cook for 1-2 minutes until fragrant.

5. Add the blackberries, balsamic vinegar, honey, and Dijon mustard. Bring the mixture to a simmer and cook for 5-7 minutes, stirring occasionally, until the sauce has thickened slightly.

6. Remove the skillet from heat and stir in the butter until melted and incorporated.

7. Slice the duck breasts and arrange on plates. Spoon the warm blackberry sauce over the top.

8. Garnish with fresh thyme sprigs.

Serve the pan-seared duck immediately with the rich, sweet blackberry sauce. The combination of the crispy duck skin, juicy meat, and tangy-sweet sauce makes for an elegant and romantic date night meal.

Pair it with a glass of red wine, a simple salad, and some crusty bread for a complete and indulgent dinner.

What are the critical points in the recipe (e.g., temperature control, timing)?

What is the total cooking time, including prep time?

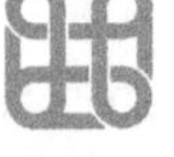 Prep Time : _________________

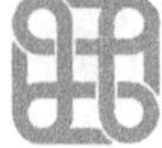 Cook Time : _________________

Servings   : _________________

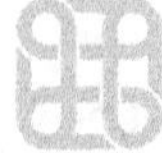 ## Ingredients:

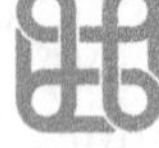
- 8 oz fettuccine or linguine pasta
- 2 tbsp unsalted butter
- 2 cloves garlic, minced
- 1 cup heavy cream
- 1/2 cup freshly grated Parmesan cheese
- 2 tsp white truffle oil
- 1 tsp lemon zest
- Salt and pepper to taste
- Chopped parsley for garnish

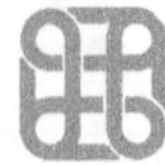
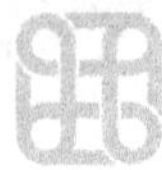

Is the recipe easy to follow?

30. Truffle pasta

Procedure:

1. Bring a large pot of salted water to a boil. Cook the pasta according to package instructions until al dente. Drain and set aside.

2. In a large skillet, melt the butter over medium heat. Add the garlic and cook for 1 minute until fragrant.

3. Pour in the heavy cream and bring to a gentle simmer. Cook for 2-3 minutes, stirring frequently, until the sauce has thickened slightly.

4. Remove the skillet from heat and stir in the Parmesan cheese until melted and smooth.

5. Add the cooked pasta, truffle oil, and lemon zest to the sauce. Toss to coat the pasta evenly.

6. Season with salt and pepper to taste.

7. Serve the truffle pasta immediately, garnished with chopped parsley.

For an extra special touch, you can shave some fresh black truffles over the top of the pasta just before serving.

This rich and decadent truffle pasta is the perfect romantic meal for a date night. The creamy sauce infused with the earthy aroma of truffles creates an indulgent and luxurious dish. Pair it with a glass of white wine, a simple salad, and some crusty bread for a complete and impressive date night dinner.

What is the total cooking time, including prep time?

Prep Time : ________________

Cook Time : ________________

Servings   : ________________

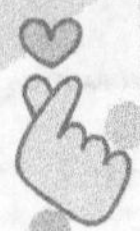

Ingredients:

- 1 lb beef tenderloin, cut into 1-inch cubes
- 2 tbsp olive oil
- 1 onion, diced
- 8 oz cremini mushrooms, sliced
- 2 cloves garlic, minced
- 1 cup beef broth
- 1/2 cup dry white wine
- 2 tbsp Dijon mustard
- 1 cup sour cream
- 2 tbsp fresh parsley, chopped
- Salt and pepper to taste
- Cooked egg noodles, for serving

Is the recipe easy to follow?

31. Beef stroganoff

Procedure:

1. Season the beef cubes generously with salt and pepper.

2. Heat the olive oil in a large skillet over medium-high heat. Working in batches if needed, sear the beef on all sides until browned, about 2-3 minutes per side. Transfer the seared beef to a plate.

3. Reduce the heat to medium and add the onions to the skillet. Cook for 5 minutes until softened.

4. Add the mushrooms and garlic and cook for 3-4 minutes more.

5. Pour in the beef broth and white wine. Use a wooden spoon to scrape up any browned bits from the bottom of the pan.

6. Stir in the Dijon mustard and sour cream until well combined.

7. Return the seared beef and any accumulated juices to the skillet. Bring the mixture to a simmer and cook for 10-15 minutes, until the beef is tender.

8. Remove from heat and stir in the chopped parsley. Taste and adjust seasoning with salt and pepper as needed.

9. Serve the beef stroganoff immediately over cooked egg noodles.

This classic beef stroganoff is an elegant and comforting dish perfect for a romantic date night. The tender beef in the rich, creamy sauce is truly indulgent. Pair it with a glass of red wine and some crusty bread for a complete and impressive meal.

What is the total cooking time, including prep time?

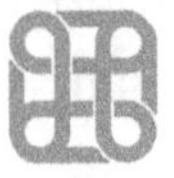 Prep Time : ________________

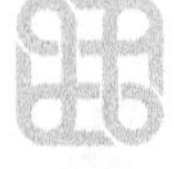 Cook Time : ________________

Servings : ________________

Ingredients:

- 6 bell peppers (mix of red, yellow, orange)
- 1 lb ground beef or ground turkey
- 1 onion, diced
- 3 cloves garlic, minced
- 1 cup cooked rice
- 1 (14.5 oz) can diced tomatoes
- 1 tsp dried oregano
- 1 tsp dried basil
- Salt and pepper to taste
- 1 cup shredded mozzarella cheese

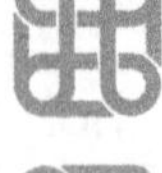
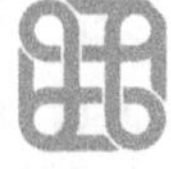
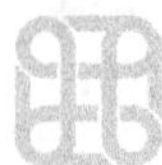

Is the recipe easy to follow?

32. Stuffed bell peppers

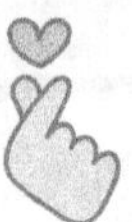

Procedure:

1. Preheat oven to 375°F.

2. Cut the tops off the bell peppers and remove the seeds and membranes. Place the peppers in a baking dish.

3. In a large skillet over medium heat, cook the ground beef or turkey until browned and crumbled, 5-7 minutes. Drain any excess fat.

4. Add the onion and garlic to the skillet and cook for 2-3 minutes until softened.

5. Stir in the cooked rice, diced tomatoes, oregano, basil, salt, and pepper. Cook for 5 minutes, allowing the flavors to meld.

6. Stuff the mixture into the hollowed-out bell peppers, packing it in tightly.

7. Top each stuffed pepper with shredded mozzarella cheese.

8. Cover the baking dish with foil and bake for 30 minutes.

9. Remove the foil and bake for an additional 10-15 minutes, until the peppers are tender and the cheese is melted and bubbly.

10. Serve the stuffed peppers warm, garnished with fresh parsley if desired.

These stuffed bell peppers make a delicious and healthy main dish. The combination of savory ground meat, rice, tomatoes, and melted cheese is so satisfying. You can customize the filling with different herbs, spices, or vegetables to your liking.

What is the total cooking time, including prep time?

Prep Time : _______________

Cook Time : _______________

Servings   : _______________

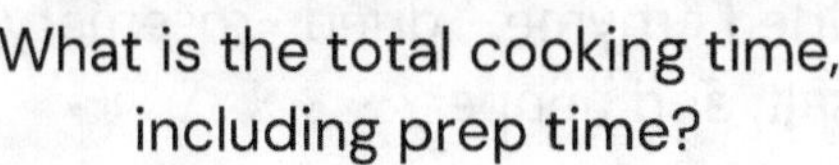

Ingredients:

- 8 oz linguine or fettuccine pasta
- 1 lb shrimp, peeled and deveined
- 3 tbsp olive oil
- 4 cloves garlic, minced
- 1/4 cup dry white wine
- 1/4 cup freshly squeezed lemon juice (about 2 lemons)
- 1/4 cup heavy cream
- 1/4 cup grated Parmesan cheese
- 2 tbsp chopped fresh parsley
- Salt and pepper to taste

Is the recipe easy to follow?

33. Lemon garlic shrimp pasta

Procedure:

1. Bring a large pot of salted water to a boil. Cook the pasta according to package instructions until al dente. Drain and set aside.

2. In a large skillet, heat the olive oil over medium-high heat. Add the shrimp and garlic and cook for 2-3 minutes, stirring frequently, until the shrimp start to turn pink.

3. Pour in the white wine and lemon juice. Let the mixture simmer for 2-3 minutes, allowing the sauce to reduce slightly.

4. Reduce the heat to low and stir in the heavy cream. Cook for 1-2 minutes, stirring constantly, until the sauce thickens.

5. Remove the skillet from heat and stir in the cooked pasta, Parmesan cheese, and parsley. Toss to combine everything evenly.

6. Season with salt and pepper to taste.

7. Serve the lemon garlic shrimp pasta immediately, garnished with extra parsley if desired.

The bright, zesty flavors of the lemon and garlic pair beautifully with the tender shrimp and creamy sauce. This pasta dish is perfect for a quick and easy weeknight meal, but it's also elegant enough for a special date night dinner.

Serve it with a crisp white wine, a fresh salad, and some crusty bread for a complete and satisfying meal.

What is the total cooking time, including prep time?

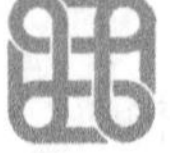
Prep Time : _______________

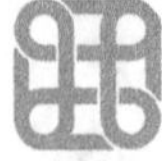
Cook Time : _______________

Servings : _______________

Ingredients:

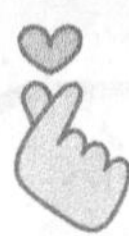

- 4 Cornish game hens (about 1-1.5 lbs each)
- 4 tbsp unsalted butter, softened
- 2 tsp dried thyme
- 1 tsp dried rosemary
- 1 tsp garlic powder
- Salt and pepper to taste
- 1 lemon, cut into wedges
- Fresh thyme and rosemary sprigs for garnish

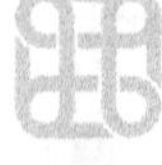
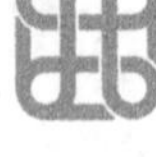
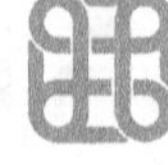

Is the recipe easy to follow?

34. Roasted Cornish game hens

Procedure:

1. Preheat oven to 400°F. Line a large baking sheet with parchment paper.

2. In a small bowl, mix together the softened butter, dried thyme, dried rosemary, garlic powder, salt, and pepper.

3. Pat the Cornish game hens dry with paper towels. Gently loosen the skin on each hen and spread about 1 tbsp of the seasoned butter under the skin, massaging it to distribute evenly.

4. Rub the remaining seasoned butter all over the outside of the hens. Season the hens generously with additional salt and pepper.

5. Arrange the hens breast-side up on the prepared baking sheet. Tuck the lemon wedges around the hens.

6. Roast for 45-55 minutes, until the internal temperature reaches 165°F. Baste the hens with the pan juices halfway through cooking.

7. Let the hens rest for 5-10 minutes before serving.

8. Garnish the roasted Cornish game hens with fresh thyme and rosemary sprigs. Serve with the roasted lemon wedges.

These elegant Cornish game hens make a beautiful and impressive main dish. The herb-butter basting keeps the meat moist and flavorful. Serve them with roasted potatoes, a fresh salad, and a glass of white wine for a complete and romantic dinner.

What is the total cooking time, including prep time?

Prep Time : ___________________

Cook Time : ___________________

Servings : ___________________

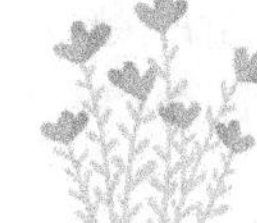

Ingredients:

- 2 medium zucchini, sliced into 1/4-inch rounds
- 2 medium yellow squash, sliced into 1/4-inch rounds
- 1 large eggplant, sliced into 1/4-inch rounds
- 1 large onion, thinly sliced
- 3 cloves garlic, minced
- 2 tbsp olive oil
- 1 tsp dried thyme
- 1 tsp dried oregano
- Salt and pepper to taste
- 1 cup shredded Gruyère or Parmesan cheese

Is the recipe easy to follow?

35. Vegetable tian

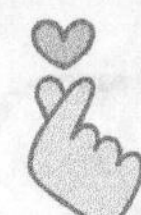

Procedure:

1. Preheat oven to 375°F. Grease a 9x13 inch baking dish.

2. In a large bowl, combine the zucchini, yellow squash, eggplant, onion, and garlic. Drizzle with the olive oil and sprinkle with the thyme, oregano, salt, and pepper. Toss to coat the vegetables evenly.

3. Arrange the vegetable slices vertically in the prepared baking dish, overlapping them slightly.

4. Cover the dish with foil and bake for 40 minutes.

5. Remove the foil and sprinkle the shredded cheese over the top of the vegetables.

6. Return the dish to the oven and bake for an additional 20-25 minutes, until the vegetables are tender and the cheese is melted and lightly browned.

7. Let the tian cool for 5-10 minutes before serving.

This colorful vegetable tian makes a beautiful and delicious side dish or vegetarian main course. The layered slices of zucchini, squash, eggplant, and onion create a stunning presentation. The herbs and melted cheese add wonderful flavor.

Serve the tian warm, garnished with fresh thyme or parsley if desired. It pairs well with roasted meats, grilled fish, or a simple salad for a complete meal.

What is the total cooking time, including prep time?

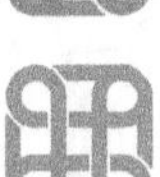
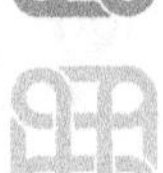
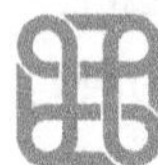
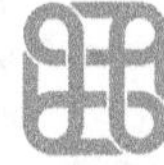

Prep Time : _______________

Cook Time : _______________

Servings   : _______________

Ingredients:

- 4 ahi tuna steaks, about 6 oz each
- 2 tbsp olive oil
- 2 tsp sesame seeds
- 1 tsp black pepper
- 1 tsp salt
- 2 tbsp soy sauce
- 1 tbsp rice vinegar
- 1 tsp honey
- 1 tsp sesame oil
- 2 tbsp chopped green onions, for garnish

Is the recipe easy to follow?

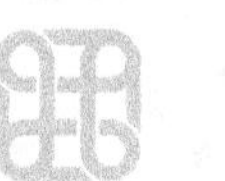

36. Seared ahi tuna steaks

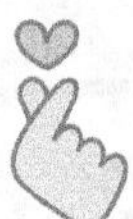

Procedure:

1. Pat the tuna steaks dry with paper towels and season both sides generously with the sesame seeds, black pepper, and salt.

2. Heat the olive oil in a large skillet or grill pan over high heat.

3. When the oil is very hot, add the tuna steaks and sear for 1-2 minutes per side, until the outside is nicely browned but the center is still pink and rare.

4. Transfer the seared tuna steaks to a cutting board and let rest for 2-3 minutes.

5. In a small bowl, whisk together the soy sauce, rice vinegar, honey, and sesame oil to make the dipping sauce.

6. Slice the tuna steaks into 1/2-inch thick slices. Arrange the slices on a serving platter and drizzle with the dipping sauce.

7. Garnish the seared ahi tuna with the chopped green onions.

Serve the seared ahi tuna immediately, with extra dipping sauce on the side. The tuna should be rare to medium-rare in the center for the best texture and flavor.

This dish makes an elegant and impressive main course, perfect for a special occasion or date night. The combination of the seared, peppery tuna and the sweet-savory dipping sauce is simply delicious.

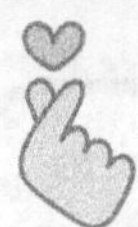

What is the total cooking time, including prep time?

Prep Time : _______________

Cook Time : _______________

Servings   : _______________

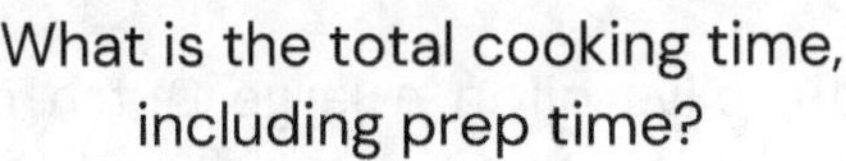

Ingredients:

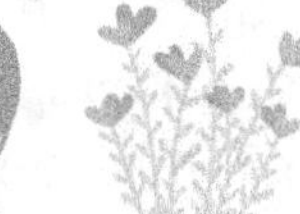

- 4 medium zucchini, halved lengthwise
- 1 lb ground turkey or ground beef
- 1 onion, diced
- 3 cloves garlic, minced
- 1 cup cooked rice
- 1 (14.5 oz) can diced tomatoes
- 1 tsp dried oregano
- 1 tsp dried basil
- Salt and pepper to taste
- 1 cup shredded mozzarella cheese

Is the recipe easy to follow?

37. Stuffed zucchini boats

1. Preheat oven to 375°F. Lightly grease a baking dish.

2. Scoop out the flesh from the center of each zucchini half, leaving about 1/4 inch of zucchini along the sides and bottom to create "boats". Finely chop the scooped out zucchini flesh.

3. In a large skillet over medium heat, cook the ground turkey or beef until browned and crumbled, 5-7 minutes. Drain any excess fat.

4. Add the diced onion, minced garlic, and chopped zucchini flesh to the skillet. Cook for 3-4 minutes until the vegetables are softened.

5. Stir in the cooked rice, diced tomatoes, oregano, basil, salt, and pepper. Cook for 5 minutes, allowing the flavors to meld.

6. Arrange the zucchini boats in the prepared baking dish. Spoon the meat and rice mixture evenly into the zucchini boats.

7. Top each stuffed zucchini boat with shredded mozzarella cheese.

8. Bake for 25-30 minutes, until the zucchini is tender and the cheese is melted and bubbly.

9. Serve the stuffed zucchini boats warm, garnished with fresh basil if desired.

These stuffed zucchini boats make a delicious and healthy main dish or side. The flavorful filling of ground meat, rice, and tomatoes complements the tender zucchini perfectly. Top it with melted cheese for an extra indulgent touch.

What is the total cooking time, including prep time?

Prep Time : _______________

Cook Time : _______________

Servings   : _______________

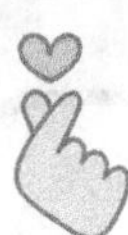

Ingredients:

- 3 lbs beef short ribs, cut into individual ribs
- 2 tbsp olive oil
- 1 onion, diced
- 3 carrots, peeled and diced
- 3 celery stalks, diced
- 4 garlic cloves, minced
- 2 cups red wine
- 2 cups beef broth
- 2 bay leaves
- 2 sprigs fresh thyme
- 1 tsp dried oregano
- Salt and pepper to taste
- Chopped parsley for garnish

Is the recipe easy to follow?

38. Beef short ribs

Procedure:

1. Preheat oven to 325°F.

2. Pat the short ribs dry and season generously with salt and pepper.

3. Heat the olive oil in a large Dutch oven or heavy-bottomed pot over medium-high heat. Working in batches if needed, sear the short ribs on all sides until deeply browned, about 3-4 minutes per side. Transfer the seared ribs to a plate.

4. Reduce the heat to medium and add the onion, carrots, celery, and garlic to the pot. Cook for 5-7 minutes, stirring occasionally, until the vegetables are softened.

5. Pour in the red wine and use a wooden spoon to scrape up any browned bits from the bottom of the pot. Allow the wine to simmer for 2-3 minutes.

6. Return the seared short ribs to the pot and add the beef broth, bay leaves, thyme, and oregano. Bring the liquid to a simmer.

7. Cover the pot and transfer to the preheated oven. Braise the short ribs for 2.5 to 3 hours, until the meat is very tender and falling off the bone.

8. Remove the pot from the oven. Transfer the short ribs to a serving platter.

9. Discard the bay leaves and thyme sprigs. Taste the braising liquid and season with additional salt and pepper as needed.

10. Serve the braised short ribs warm, garnished with chopped parsley. Spoon some of the braising liquid over the top.

What is the total cooking time, including prep time?

Prep Time : _______________

Cook Time : _______________

Servings : _______________

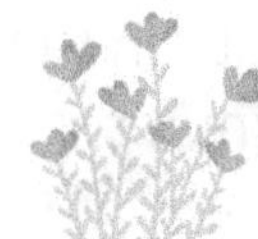

Ingredients:

- 1 medium eggplant, cut into 1-inch cubes
- 1 medium zucchini, sliced into 1/2-inch rounds
- 1 yellow squash, sliced into 1/2-inch rounds
- 1 red bell pepper, diced
- 1 onion, diced
- 3 cloves garlic, minced
- 2 tbsp olive oil
- 1 (14.5 oz) can diced tomatoes
- 2 tbsp tomato paste
- 1 tsp dried thyme
- 1 tsp dried oregano
- Salt and pepper to taste
- Chopped fresh basil for garnish

39. Ratatouille

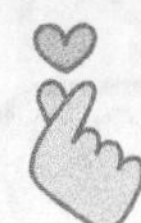

Procedure:

1. Preheat oven to 400°F. Line a large baking sheet with parchment paper.

2. In a large bowl, toss the eggplant, zucchini, yellow squash, bell pepper, onion, and garlic with the olive oil. Season with salt and pepper.

3. Spread the vegetables in a single layer on the prepared baking sheet. Roast for 25-30 minutes, stirring halfway, until the vegetables are tender and lightly browned.

4. In a large saucepan, combine the roasted vegetables, diced tomatoes, tomato paste, thyme, and oregano. Stir to combine.

5. Bring the mixture to a simmer over medium heat. Reduce heat to low and let the ratatouille simmer for 15-20 minutes, stirring occasionally, until the flavors have melded.

6. Taste and adjust seasoning with salt and pepper as needed.

7. Serve the ratatouille warm, garnished with chopped fresh basil.

This classic French vegetable stew is full of vibrant flavors and colors. The roasting step brings out the natural sweetness of the vegetables. Serve ratatouille as a side dish or a vegetarian main course. It pairs well with crusty bread, grilled meats, or pasta.

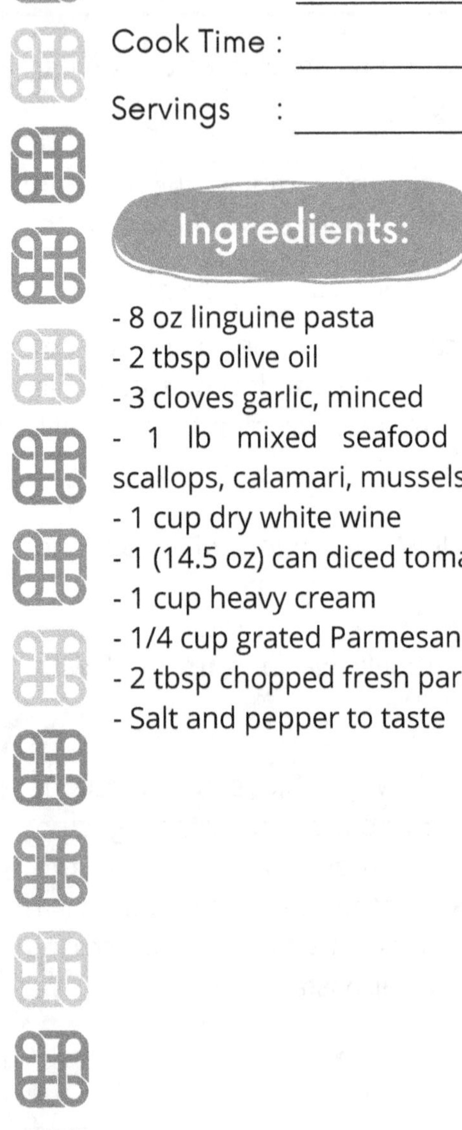

Prep Time : ________________

Cook Time : ________________

Servings : ________________

Ingredients:

- 8 oz linguine pasta
- 2 tbsp olive oil
- 3 cloves garlic, minced
- 1 lb mixed seafood (shrimp, scallops, calamari, mussels)
- 1 cup dry white wine
- 1 (14.5 oz) can diced tomatoes
- 1 cup heavy cream
- 1/4 cup grated Parmesan cheese
- 2 tbsp chopped fresh parsley
- Salt and pepper to taste

Is the recipe easy to follow?

40. Seafood linguine

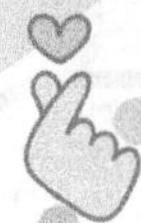

Procedure:

1. Bring a large pot of salted water to a boil. Cook the linguine according to package instructions until al dente. Drain and set aside.

2. In a large skillet, heat the olive oil over medium heat. Add the minced garlic and cook for 1 minute until fragrant.

3. Add the mixed seafood to the skillet. Cook for 2-3 minutes, stirring occasionally, until the seafood starts to turn opaque.

4. Pour in the white wine and let it simmer for 2-3 minutes, allowing the alcohol to cook off.

5. Stir in the diced tomatoes and their juices. Bring the mixture to a simmer.

6. Reduce heat to low and stir in the heavy cream. Cook for 3-5 minutes, stirring frequently, until the sauce has thickened slightly.

7. Remove the skillet from heat and stir in the cooked linguine, Parmesan cheese, and chopped parsley. Toss to coat the pasta evenly.

8. Season the seafood linguine with salt and pepper to taste.

9. Serve the seafood linguine immediately, garnished with extra parsley if desired.

This seafood linguine is an elegant and flavorful pasta dish. The combination of tender seafood, creamy tomato sauce, and al dente linguine makes for a truly delicious meal. Pair it with a crisp white wine and a fresh salad for a complete and satisfying dinner.

What is the total cooking time,
including prep time?

Prep Time : _______________

Cook Time : _______________

Servings   : _______________

Ingredients:

- 1 (3-4 lb) pork rack (also called pork crown roast)
- 2 tbsp olive oil
- 2 tsp garlic powder
- 2 tsp dried thyme
- 1 tsp salt
- 1/2 tsp black pepper
- 1/2 cup apple cider or apple juice
- 2 tbsp Dijon mustard
- 2 tbsp honey

Is the recipe easy to follow?

41. Roasted rack of pork

Procedure:

1. Preheat oven to 400°F.

2. Pat the pork rack dry with paper towels. Use kitchen string to tie the roast into a circle, securing the ends together.

3. In a small bowl, mix together the olive oil, garlic powder, dried thyme, salt, and pepper. Rub this seasoning mixture all over the outside of the pork rack.

4. Place the pork rack, fat-side up, in a large roasting pan or baking dish. Pour the apple cider or juice into the bottom of the pan.

5. Roast the pork for 30 minutes.

6. In a small bowl, whisk together the Dijon mustard and honey. Brush this glaze all over the top and sides of the pork.

7. Continue roasting the pork for 45-60 minutes more, until the internal temperature reaches 145°F.

8. Transfer the roasted pork rack to a cutting board and let rest for 15 minutes before slicing.

9. Slice the pork between the bones to create individual chops. Serve warm, drizzled with any pan juices.

This impressive roasted rack of pork makes a wonderful main dish for a special occasion or holiday meal. The savory herb seasoning and sweet honey-mustard glaze create a delicious flavor profile. Serve it with roasted vegetables, mashed potatoes, and a crisp white wine for a complete and elegant dinner.

What is the total cooking time, including prep time?

Prep Time : _______________

Cook Time : _______________

Servings   : _______________

Ingredients:

- 1 jar (16 oz) grape leaves, drained and rinsed
- 1 cup cooked rice
- 1 onion, finely chopped
- 2 cloves garlic, minced
- 1/2 cup chopped parsley
- 1/4 cup chopped mint
- 1 tbsp olive oil
- Juice of 1 lemon
- Salt and pepper to taste

For the Lemon Sauce:
- 1/2 cup olive oil
- 1/4 cup lemon juice
- 2 cloves garlic, minced
- 1 tsp dried oregano
- Salt and pepper to taste

Is the recipe easy to follow?

42. Vegetarian stuffed grape leaves

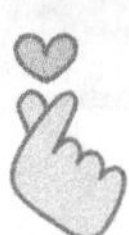

Procedure:

1. In a medium bowl, mix together the cooked rice, onion, garlic, parsley, mint, 1 tbsp olive oil, and lemon juice. Season with salt and pepper.

2. Carefully unroll the grape leaves, keeping them intact. Place about 1-2 tbsp of the rice filling near the stem end of each leaf. Fold the sides over the filling, then tightly roll up the leaf.

3. Arrange the stuffed grape leaves seam-side down in a large pot or baking dish.

4. In a small bowl, whisk together the ingredients for the lemon sauce. Pour the sauce over the stuffed grape leaves, making sure they are all coated.

5. Cover the pot or dish and refrigerate for at least 2 hours, or up to 24 hours, to allow the flavors to meld.

6. When ready to serve, remove the grape leaves from the refrigerator and let sit at room temperature for 30 minutes.

7. Serve the chilled stuffed grape leaves drizzled with any remaining lemon sauce. Garnish with extra parsley if desired.

These vegetarian stuffed grape leaves make a delightful appetizer or light main course. The tangy lemon sauce complements the savory rice and herb filling perfectly. They can be made ahead of time, making them ideal for entertaining.

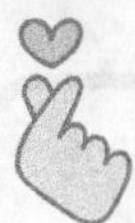

What is the total cooking time, including prep time?

Prep Time : _________________

Cook Time : _________________

Servings   : _________________

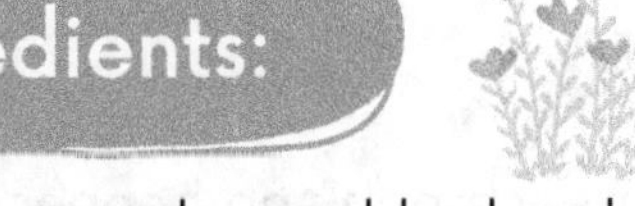

Ingredients:

- 2 lbs fresh mussels, scrubbed and debearded
- 2 tbsp unsalted butter
- 1 shallot, finely chopped
- 3 garlic cloves, minced
- 1 cup dry white wine
- 1/2 cup heavy cream
- 2 tbsp chopped fresh parsley
- Salt and pepper to taste
- Crusty bread, for serving

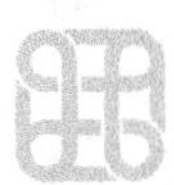
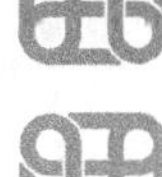
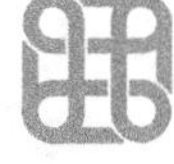
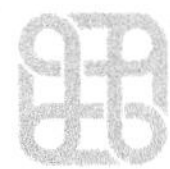

Is the recipe easy to follow?

43. Moules marinières

1. Rinse the mussels under cold running water, scrubbing off any dirt or debris. Pull off and discard any beards (the fibrous strings attached to the shells).

2. In a large pot or Dutch oven, melt the butter over medium heat. Add the shallot and garlic and cook for 1-2 minutes until fragrant.

3. Pour in the white wine and bring to a simmer. Add the mussels, cover the pot, and cook for 5-7 minutes, shaking the pot occasionally, until the mussels have opened up.

4. Discard any mussels that did not open.

5. Stir in the heavy cream and chopped parsley. Season with salt and pepper to taste.

6. Serve the mussels immediately in shallow bowls, with the sauce spooned over the top. Provide crusty bread for dipping in the sauce.

Tips:
- Make sure to discard any mussels that are cracked or won't close when tapped.
- Serve with a crisp white wine for the full French bistro experience.
- For a heartier meal, serve the mussels over pasta or with fries on the side.

Enjoy this classic French seafood dish!

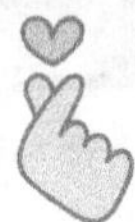

What is the total cooking time, including prep time?

Prep Time : _______________

Cook Time : _______________

Servings   : _______________

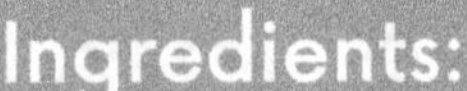

Ingredients:

- 6 large poblano peppers
- 1 lb ground beef or ground turkey
- 1 onion, diced
- 3 cloves garlic, minced
- 1 cup cooked rice
- 1 cup shredded cheddar or Monterey Jack cheese
- 1 tsp cumin
- 1 tsp chili powder
- Salt and pepper to taste
- Olive oil

Is the recipe easy to follow?

44. Stuffed poblano peppers

1. Preheat oven to 375°F.

2. Slice the poblano peppers in half lengthwise and remove the seeds and membranes. Place the pepper halves in a baking dish.

3. In a skillet over medium heat, cook the ground beef or turkey with the onion and garlic until browned and cooked through, 5-7 minutes. Drain any excess fat.

4. Stir in the cooked rice, 1/2 cup of the shredded cheese, cumin, chili powder, salt and pepper.

5. Stuff each poblano pepper half with the beef and rice mixture, packing it in tightly.

6. Drizzle the stuffed peppers lightly with olive oil.

7. Bake for 20-25 minutes until the peppers are tender.

8. Remove from oven and top with the remaining 1/2 cup shredded cheese.

9. Return to oven for 5 more minutes until the cheese is melted.

10. Serve hot. Enjoy!

What is the total cooking time, including prep time?

Prep Time : ___________________

Cook Time : ___________________

Servings : ___________________

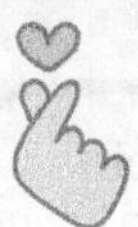

Ingredients:

- 4 boneless, skinless chicken breasts
- 4 slices Swiss cheese
- 4 slices ham or prosciutto
- 1/2 cup all-purpose flour
- 2 eggs, beaten
- 1 cup breadcrumbs
- 2 tbsp butter
- 2 tbsp olive oil

For the Sauce:
- 1 cup chicken broth
- 1/2 cup heavy cream
- 2 tbsp Dijon mustard
- 1 tbsp lemon juice
- Salt and pepper to taste

Is the recipe easy to follow?

45. Chicken cordon bleu

Procedure:

1. Preheat oven to 400°F.

2. Pound the chicken breasts between two sheets of plastic wrap or wax paper until they are about 1/4 inch thick.

3. Place a slice of Swiss cheese and a slice of ham on each chicken breast. Fold the chicken over the filling and secure with toothpicks.

4. Set up a breading station with the flour, beaten eggs, and breadcrumbs in separate shallow dishes.

5. Dredge the stuffed chicken breasts in the flour, then dip in the egg, and finally coat in the breadcrumbs.

6. In a large skillet, heat the butter and olive oil over medium-high heat.

7. Carefully add the breaded chicken breasts and cook for 2-3 minutes per side until golden brown.

8. Transfer the chicken to a baking sheet and bake for 15-20 minutes until the chicken is cooked through.

For the Sauce:
1. In a small saucepan, whisk together the chicken broth, heavy cream, Dijon mustard, and lemon juice.
2. Season with salt and pepper.
3. Bring the sauce to a simmer and cook for 5-7 minutes until slightly thickened.

Serve the chicken cordon bleu warm, drizzled with the creamy mustard sauce.

What is the total cooking time, including prep time?

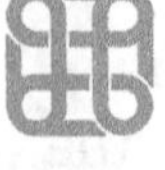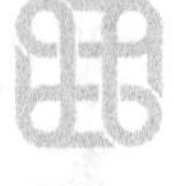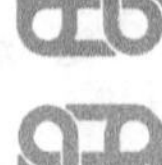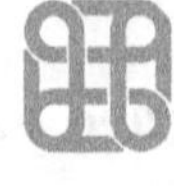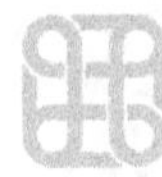

Prep Time : _______________

Cook Time : _______________

Servings   : _______________

Ingredients:

- 2 medium eggplants, sliced lengthwise into 1/4-inch thick slices
- Olive oil
- Salt and pepper
- 1 cup ricotta cheese
- 1 cup shredded mozzarella cheese
- 1/2 cup grated Parmesan cheese
- 1 egg, beaten
- 2 cloves garlic, minced
- 1/4 cup chopped fresh basil
- 1 cup marinara sauce
- Fresh basil leaves for garnish

Is the recipe easy to follow?

46. Eggplant involtini

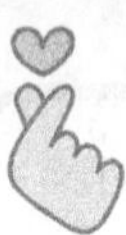

Procedure:

1. Preheat oven to 400°F.

2. Arrange the eggplant slices in a single layer on baking sheets. Brush both sides with olive oil and season with salt and pepper.

3. Bake the eggplant for 15-20 minutes, flipping halfway, until softened and lightly browned. Allow to cool slightly.

4. In a medium bowl, mix together the ricotta, mozzarella, Parmesan, egg, garlic, and chopped basil. Season with salt and pepper.

5. Spread about 2-3 tablespoons of the cheese mixture onto the wide end of each eggplant slice. Carefully roll up the eggplant around the filling.

6. Arrange the eggplant rolls seam-side down in a baking dish. Pour the marinara sauce over the top.

7. Bake for 20-25 minutes, until the cheese is melted and bubbly.

8. Garnish with fresh basil leaves before serving.

Serve the eggplant involtini warm, with extra marinara sauce if desired. Enjoy!

What is the total cooking time, including prep time?

Prep Time : ______________

Cook Time : ______________

Servings   : ______________

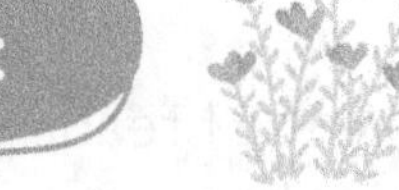

Ingredients:

- 8 oz beef tenderloin, trimmed of fat and silver skin
- 2 tbsp olive oil
- 1 tsp lemon zest
- 1 tbsp lemon juice
- 1 tsp Dijon mustard
- Salt and freshly ground black pepper
- Arugula or mixed greens
- Shaved Parmesan cheese
- Capers (optional)
- Lemon wedges, for serving

Is the recipe easy to follow?

47. Beef carpaccio

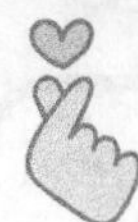

Procedure:

1. Place the beef tenderloin in the freezer for 30-60 minutes to firm up slightly, making it easier to slice.

2. In a small bowl, whisk together the olive oil, lemon zest, lemon juice, and Dijon mustard. Season with a pinch of salt and pepper.

3. Remove the tenderloin from the freezer and, using a very sharp knife, slice it into paper-thin slices. Arrange the slices in a single layer on a large plate or platter.

4. Drizzle the lemon-mustard dressing evenly over the beef slices, making sure to coat them all.

5. Cover the plate with plastic wrap and refrigerate for 30 minutes to 1 hour, allowing the flavors to meld.

6. To serve, arrange a bed of arugula or mixed greens on each plate. Top with the chilled beef carpaccio slices.

7. Garnish with shaved Parmesan cheese and capers, if desired.

8. Serve immediately with lemon wedges on the side.

This beef carpaccio makes an elegant and romantic starter or light main course for a date night. The thinly sliced raw beef is delicately flavored with the bright lemon-mustard dressing. The peppery arugula and salty Parmesan provide a perfect contrast.

Pair the carpaccio with a crisp white wine or sparkling wine for a truly indulgent and impressive date night meal.

What is the total cooking time, including prep time?

Prep Time : _______________

Cook Time : _______________

Servings   : _______________

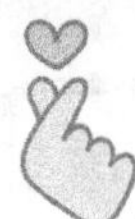

Ingredients:

- 4 medium artichokes
- 1 cup breadcrumbs
- 1/2 cup grated Parmesan cheese
- 1/4 cup chopped fresh parsley
- 2 cloves garlic, minced
- 2 tbsp olive oil, plus more for drizzling
- 1 lemon, cut into wedges
- Salt and pepper to taste

For the Stuffing:
- 1 cup cooked rice
- 1/2 cup chopped onion
- 2 cloves garlic, minced
- 1/4 cup chopped fresh parsley
- 2 tbsp olive oil
- Salt and pepper to taste

Is the recipe easy to follow?

48. Stuffed artichokes

Procedure:

1. Prepare the artichokes:
- Trim the stems and bottom leaves of the artichokes. Use kitchen shears to snip off the thorny tips of the leaves.
- Use a sharp knife to slice off the top 1-2 inches of the artichokes.
- Use a spoon to scoop out the fuzzy choke in the center, being careful not to remove the heart.

2. Make the stuffing:
- In a bowl, mix together the cooked rice, onion, garlic, parsley, olive oil, salt and pepper.

3. Make the breadcrumb topping:
- In another bowl, combine the breadcrumbs, Parmesan, parsley, garlic, and 2 tbsp olive oil. Season with salt and pepper.

4. Stuff the artichokes:
- Spoon the rice stuffing into the center of each artichoke, packing it in tightly.
- Top each stuffed artichoke with the breadcrumb mixture, pressing it down gently.

5. Arrange the stuffed artichokes in a baking dish and drizzle with a bit of olive oil.

6. Bake at 375°F for 45-60 minutes, until the artichokes are tender when pierced with a knife.

7. Serve the stuffed artichokes warm, with lemon wedges on the side.

Enjoy this delicious and impressive stuffed artichoke dish!

What is the total cooking time, including prep time?

Prep Time : _______________

Cook Time : _______________

Servings : _______________

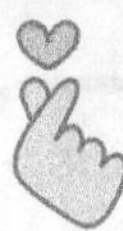

Ingredients:

- 1 lb asparagus, tough ends trimmed
- 8 oz thinly sliced prosciutto
- 2 tbsp olive oil
- 1 tbsp balsamic glaze (or balsamic vinegar)
- Salt and pepper to taste

Is the recipe easy to follow?

49. Prosciutto-wrapped asparagus

Procedure:

1. Preheat oven to 400°F. Line a baking sheet with parchment paper.

2. Wrap each asparagus spear with a slice of prosciutto, overlapping the ends slightly to secure it.

3. Arrange the prosciutto-wrapped asparagus in a single layer on the prepared baking sheet.

4. Drizzle the asparagus with the olive oil and balsamic glaze. Season with salt and pepper.

5. Roast for 12-15 minutes, until the asparagus is tender and the prosciutto is crispy.

6. Serve the prosciutto-wrapped asparagus immediately, while hot.

Tips:
- Choose thin, young asparagus spears for the best texture.
- You can use toothpicks to secure the prosciutto if needed.
- For extra flavor, try adding a sprinkle of grated Parmesan cheese or a squeeze of lemon juice.
- This makes a great appetizer or side dish.

Enjoy this simple yet elegant prosciutto-wrapped asparagus!

What is the total cooking time, including prep time?

Prep Time : _______________

Cook Time : _______________

Servings : _______________

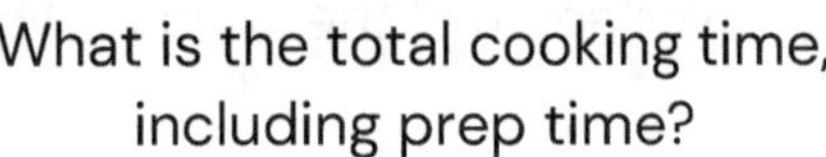

Ingredients:

- 8 oz elbow macaroni
- 2 tbsp unsalted butter
- 2 tbsp all-purpose flour
- 2 cups whole milk
- 1 cup heavy cream
- 1 tsp Dijon mustard
- 1/2 tsp paprika
- 1/4 tsp cayenne pepper
- 1 lb cooked lobster meat, chopped into bite-sized pieces
- 2 cups shredded sharp cheddar cheese
- 1 cup shredded Gruyère cheese
- Salt and pepper to taste
- Panko breadcrumbs (optional)

Is the recipe easy to follow?

50. Lobster mac and cheese

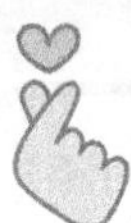

Procedure:

1. Preheat oven to 375°F. Grease a 9x13 inch baking dish.

2. Cook the macaroni according to package instructions until al dente. Drain and set aside.

3. In a large saucepan, melt the butter over medium heat. Whisk in the flour and cook for 1 minute.

4. Gradually whisk in the milk and heavy cream. Bring to a simmer and cook, stirring frequently, until thickened, about 5 minutes.

5. Remove from heat and stir in the Dijon mustard, paprika, cayenne, and 1 cup each of the cheddar and Gruyère cheeses. Season with salt and pepper.

6. Add the cooked macaroni and lobster meat to the cheese sauce and stir to combine.

7. Transfer the mac and cheese to the prepared baking dish. Top with the remaining 1 cup of cheddar and Gruyère cheeses.

8. If desired, sprinkle the top with panko breadcrumbs.

9. Bake for 20-25 minutes, until the cheese is melted and bubbly.

10. Let stand for 5 minutes before serving.

Enjoy this rich and decadent lobster mac and cheese!

What is the total cooking time, including prep time?

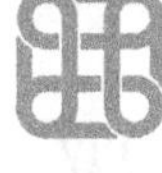 Prep Time : ___________________

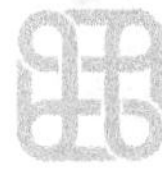 Cook Time : ___________________

Servings : ___________________

Ingredients:

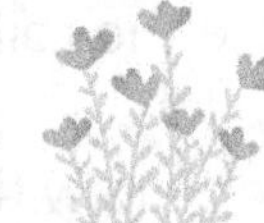

- 4 whole quail, rinsed and patted dry
- 2 tbsp olive oil
- Salt and pepper to taste
- 1 cup red grapes, halved
- 1/2 cup dry white wine
- 2 tbsp balsamic vinegar
- 2 tbsp honey
- 1 tbsp butter
- 2 tbsp chopped fresh parsley

Is the recipe easy to follow?

51. Roasted quail with grape sauce

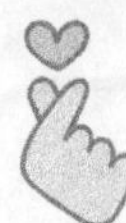

Procedure:

1. Preheat oven to 400°F.

2. Rub the quail all over with the olive oil and season generously with salt and pepper.

3. Place the quail in a roasting pan and roast for 20-25 minutes, until the juices run clear when pierced. Transfer the quail to a plate and let rest.

4. In a small saucepan, combine the grapes, wine, balsamic vinegar and honey. Bring to a simmer and cook for 5-7 minutes, until the grapes have softened and the sauce has thickened slightly.

5. Remove the saucepan from heat and stir in the butter until melted and incorporated.

6. To serve, place the roasted quail on a platter and spoon the warm grape sauce over the top. Garnish with chopped parsley.

Enjoy your tender, flavorful roasted quail with the sweet and tangy grape sauce!

What is the total cooking time, including prep time?

Prep Time : _______________

Cook Time : _______________

Servings   : _______________

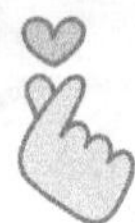

Ingredients:

- 2 cups sushi rice, cooked and cooled
- 4 sheets nori (seaweed sheets)
- 1 avocado, sliced
- 1 cucumber, julienned
- 1 carrot, julienned
- 1 red bell pepper, julienned
- 1 cup cooked edamame, shelled
- 1/2 cup pickled ginger
- 2 tbsp sesame seeds
- Soy sauce, for serving
- Wasabi, for serving
- Pickled ginger, for serving

Is the recipe easy to follow?

52. Vegetarian sushi platter

Procedure:

1. Lay a sheet of nori on a bamboo sushi mat. Spread about 1/2 cup of the sushi rice evenly over the nori, leaving a 1-inch border at the top.

2. Arrange a few slices of avocado, cucumber, carrot and bell pepper in a line across the center of the rice.

3. Carefully roll the sushi up tightly, using the bamboo mat to help. Wet the top inch of the nori to help it seal.

4. Slice the rolled sushi into 6-8 pieces.

5. Repeat with the remaining nori sheets and fillings.

6. Arrange the sushi rolls on a platter along with the edamame, pickled ginger, and sesame seeds.

7. Serve the sushi platter with soy sauce, wasabi and extra pickled ginger on the side.

For a romantic date night, you can garnish the platter with fresh herbs, edible flowers or even a drizzle of spicy mayo. Pair with chilled sake or white wine for a complete date night experience.

Enjoy this colorful, flavorful and visually impressive vegetarian sushi platter!

What are the critical points in the recipe (e.g., temperature control, timing)?

What is the total cooking time, including prep time?

Prep Time : ______________

Cook Time : ______________

Servings   : ______________

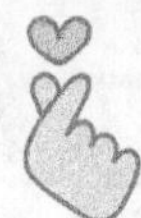

Ingredients:

- 12 littleneck or cherrystone clams, scrubbed clean
- 2 tbsp unsalted butter, softened
- 2 tbsp panko breadcrumbs
- 2 tbsp grated Parmesan cheese
- 2 tbsp finely chopped red bell pepper
- 2 tbsp finely chopped shallot
- 1 garlic clove, minced
- 1 tbsp chopped fresh parsley
- 1 tsp lemon zest
- Salt and pepper to taste

Is the recipe easy to follow?

53. Clams casino

Procedure:

1. Preheat your oven to 400°F.

2. Shuck the clams, reserving the bottom shells. Discard the top shells. Place the clams in their bottom shells on a baking sheet.

3. In a small bowl, mix together the softened butter, panko, Parmesan, bell pepper, shallot, garlic, parsley and lemon zest. Season with salt and pepper.

4. Top each clam with a generous spoonful of the breadcrumb mixture, pressing it down lightly to adhere.

5. Bake the stuffed clams for 12-15 minutes, until the topping is golden brown and the clams are cooked through.

6. Serve the clams casino immediately, while hot. You can garnish the platter with lemon wedges.

For a romantic date night, you can serve the clams casino as an appetizer or first course. Pair it with a crisp white wine like Sauvignon Blanc or Pinot Grigio.

The combination of the briny clams, crunchy topping, and bright flavors makes this an elegant and impressive dish that's perfect for an intimate dinner. Enjoy!

What is the total cooking time, including prep time?

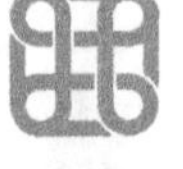
Prep Time : _______________

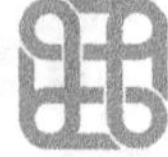
Cook Time : _______________

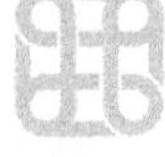
Servings   : _______________

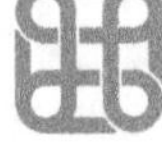

Ingredients:

- 6 medium-sized tomatoes
- 1/2 cup cooked rice
- 1/4 cup finely chopped onion
- 2 cloves garlic, minced
- 1/4 cup grated Parmesan cheese
- 2 tbsp chopped fresh basil
- 1 tbsp olive oil
- Salt and pepper to taste
- Balsamic glaze, for drizzling

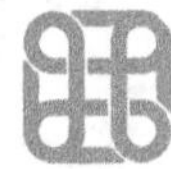
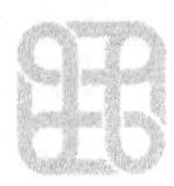

Is the recipe easy to follow?

54. Stuffed tomatoes

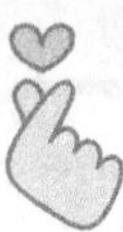

Procedure:

1. Preheat your oven to 375°F.

2. Slice the tops off the tomatoes and scoop out the insides, reserving the pulp. Finely chop the tomato pulp.

3. In a bowl, mix together the chopped tomato pulp, cooked rice, onion, garlic, Parmesan, basil, olive oil, salt and pepper.

4. Stuff the tomato shells evenly with the rice mixture.

5. Place the stuffed tomatoes in a baking dish. Bake for 20-25 minutes, until the tomatoes are softened and the filling is hot.

6. Remove from the oven and drizzle the tops of the stuffed tomatoes with balsamic glaze.

7. Serve the stuffed tomatoes warm, garnished with extra basil if desired.

For a romantic date night, you can arrange the stuffed tomatoes on a platter and serve them as an appetizer or side dish. The vibrant colors, fresh flavors, and elegant presentation make this a perfect option.

Pair the stuffed tomatoes with a light salad, crusty bread, and a glass of crisp white wine or rosé for a complete and romantic meal.

Enjoy this delicious and visually appealing stuffed tomato dish!

What is the total cooking time, including prep time?

Prep Time : _______________

Cook Time : _______________

Servings : _______________

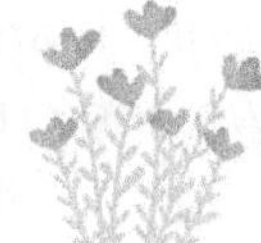

Ingredients:

- 4 veal cutlets, pounded thin
- 1/4 cup all-purpose flour
- 2 tbsp olive oil
- 2 tbsp unsalted butter
- 1/2 cup dry white wine
- 2 tbsp freshly squeezed lemon juice
- 2 tbsp capers, rinsed and drained
- 2 tbsp chopped fresh parsley
- Salt and pepper to taste

Is the recipe easy to follow?

55. Veal piccata

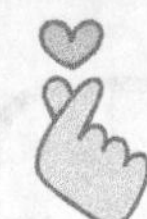

Procedure:

1. Season the veal cutlets with salt and pepper. Dredge them lightly in the flour, shaking off any excess.

2. In a large skillet, heat the olive oil and 1 tbsp of the butter over medium-high heat.

3. Working in batches if needed, add the veal cutlets to the hot pan and cook for 2-3 minutes per side, until golden brown. Transfer the cooked cutlets to a plate.

4. Add the white wine to the pan, scraping up any browned bits from the bottom. Allow the wine to simmer for 1-2 minutes.

5. Remove the pan from heat and stir in the remaining 1 tbsp of butter, lemon juice, capers and parsley. Season the sauce with salt and pepper.

6. Return the veal cutlets to the pan and spoon the sauce over the top.

7. Serve the veal piccata immediately, garnished with extra parsley if desired. Pair with roasted potatoes or a fresh salad.

For a romantic date night, you can plate the veal piccata elegantly on a platter or individual plates. The bright, tangy flavors and tender veal make this an impressive yet easy-to-prepare dish.

Accompany the veal with a crisp white wine like Pinot Grigio or Sauvignon Blanc for a complete date night meal. Enjoy!

What is the total cooking time, including prep time?

Prep Time : _________________

Cook Time : _________________

Servings   : _________________

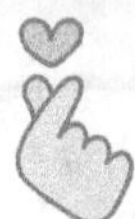

Ingredients:

- 1 cup all-purpose flour
- 1 egg, lightly beaten
- 1 cup cold soda water or club soda
- 1/2 teaspoon salt
- Assorted vegetables (such as sliced zucchini, sweet potato, bell pepper, onion, mushrooms)
- Vegetable oil for frying
- Dipping sauce (such as tentsuyu sauce, ponzu sauce, or spicy mayo)

Is the recipe easy to follow?

56. Vegetable tempura

Procedure:

1. In a large bowl, whisk together the flour, egg, soda water, and salt until just combined (do not overmix). The batter should be slightly lumpy.

2. Heat 2-3 inches of vegetable oil in a large pot or Dutch oven to 350°F.

3. Working in batches, dip the vegetable slices into the tempura batter, allowing any excess to drip off.

4. Carefully lower the battered vegetables into the hot oil and fry for 2-3 minutes until golden brown and crispy.

5. Remove the tempura with a slotted spoon and drain on a paper towel-lined plate.

6. Serve the hot tempura immediately with the dipping sauce on the side.

7. For a romantic presentation, arrange the tempura attractively on a platter and garnish with fresh herbs or lemon wedges.

The light, crispy tempura paired with the flavorful dipping sauce makes for an elegant and indulgent date night meal. Enjoy this together with your partner for a special evening.

What is the total cooking time, including prep time?

Prep Time : _______________

Cook Time : _______________

Servings   : _______________

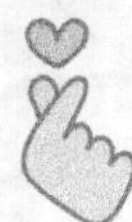

Ingredients:

- 8 oz high-quality beef tenderloin, finely chopped
- 2 egg yolks
- 2 tbsp Dijon mustard
- 2 tbsp Worcestershire sauce
- 1 tbsp capers, rinsed and chopped
- 2 tbsp finely chopped shallot
- 1 tbsp finely chopped parsley
- 1 tbsp olive oil
- Salt and freshly ground black pepper to taste
- Toasted bread or crostini, for serving

Is the recipe easy to follow?

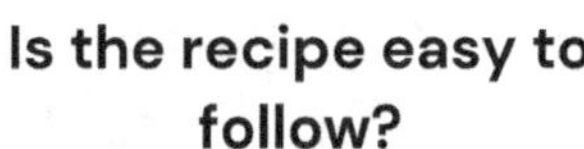
57. Beef tartare

Procedure:

1. In a medium bowl, gently mix together the chopped beef, egg yolks, Dijon, Worcestershire, capers, shallot, parsley, and olive oil until just combined. Season generously with salt and pepper.

2. Divide the beef tartare mixture evenly between 2 plates or small bowls. Use the back of a spoon to gently shape the tartare into a round mound.

3. Serve the beef tartare immediately with the toasted bread or crostini on the side. Provide small forks or spoons for guests to scoop up the tartare.

For a romantic presentation, you can garnish the tartare with a drizzle of olive oil, a sprinkle of chopped parsley, or a few capers. Serve with a crisp white wine or champagne for a truly indulgent date night meal.

The raw, high-quality beef combined with the bold flavors of the dressing makes for an elegant and intimate dining experience. Enjoy this together with your partner for a special evening.

What is the total cooking time, including prep time?

Prep Time : _______________

Cook Time : _______________

Servings : _______________

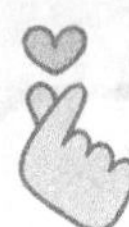

Ingredients:

- 12-16 medium-sized mushrooms, stems removed and finely chopped
- 2 tbsp olive oil
- 2 cloves garlic, minced
- 2 oz cream cheese, softened
- 1/4 cup grated Parmesan cheese
- 2 tbsp panko breadcrumbs
- 1 tbsp chopped fresh parsley
- Salt and pepper to taste

Is the recipe easy to follow?

58. Stuffed mushrooms

Procedure:

1. Preheat your oven to 375°F. Clean the mushrooms and carefully remove the stems, finely chopping them.

2. In a skillet, heat the olive oil over medium heat. Add the chopped mushroom stems and garlic. Sauté for 3-4 minutes until softened.

3. In a medium bowl, mix together the sautéed mushroom stems, cream cheese, Parmesan, panko, and parsley until well combined. Season with salt and pepper.

4. Spoon or pipe the filling into the mushroom caps, mounding it slightly on top.

5. Arrange the stuffed mushrooms on a baking sheet lined with parchment paper.

6. Bake for 12-15 minutes, until the mushrooms are tender and the filling is hot and lightly browned on top.

7. Serve the stuffed mushrooms warm, garnished with extra parsley if desired.

For a romantic presentation, you can arrange the stuffed mushrooms on a platter and serve them as an appetizer or side dish. The creamy, cheesy filling paired with the savory mushrooms makes for an indulgent and elegant date night bite.

These stuffed mushrooms can be prepared ahead of time and baked just before serving for maximum freshness. Enjoy them together with your partner for a cozy, intimate evening.

What is the total cooking time, including prep time?

Prep Time : ________________

Cook Time : ________________

Servings   : ________________

Ingredients:

- 1 lb fresh octopus, cleaned and tentacles separated
- 2 tbsp olive oil
- 2 tbsp lemon juice
- 2 cloves garlic, minced
- 1 tsp paprika
- 1/2 tsp crushed red pepper flakes
- Salt and pepper to taste
- Lemon wedges for serving

Is the recipe easy to follow?

59. Grilled octopus

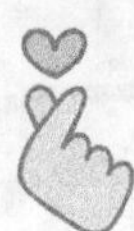

Procedure:

1. In a large bowl, combine the octopus tentacles, olive oil, lemon juice, garlic, paprika, red pepper flakes, salt, and pepper. Toss to coat the octopus evenly.

2. Preheat your grill or grill pan to medium-high heat.

3. Carefully place the octopus tentacles on the hot grill. Cook for 3-4 minutes per side, until charred and cooked through. Be gentle when flipping to prevent the octopus from falling apart.

4. Transfer the grilled octopus to a serving platter. Drizzle with any remaining marinade from the bowl.

5. Serve the grilled octopus warm, garnished with lemon wedges.

For a romantic presentation, you can arrange the octopus tentacles in an overlapping pattern on the platter. Serve with a crisp white wine or rosé for a truly indulgent date night meal.

The smoky, charred octopus paired with the bright lemon and garlic flavors makes for an elegant and flavorful dish. Enjoy this together with your partner for a special evening.

What is the total cooking time, including prep time?

Prep Time : _______________

Cook Time : _______________

Servings   : _______________

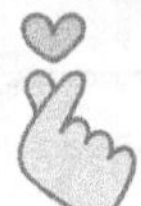

Ingredients:

- 8 oz rice paper wrappers
- 1 cup shredded cabbage
- 1 cup shredded carrots
- 1 cup thinly sliced cucumber
- 1/2 cup thinly sliced red bell pepper
- 1/2 cup thinly sliced green onions
- 1/4 cup fresh mint leaves
- 1/4 cup fresh cilantro leaves
- 2 tbsp sesame seeds
- 2 tbsp hoisin sauce
- 1 tbsp rice vinegar
- 1 tsp sesame oil
- Salt and pepper to taste

For the Dipping Sauce:
- 1/4 cup soy sauce
- 2 tbsp rice vinegar
- 1 tbsp honey
- 1 tsp sesame oil
- 1 tsp grated ginger
- 1 clove garlic, minced

Is the recipe easy to follow?

59. Grilled octopus

Procedure:

1. In a large bowl, combine the cabbage, carrots, cucumber, bell pepper, green onions, mint, cilantro, and sesame seeds.

2. In a small bowl, whisk together the hoisin sauce, rice vinegar, and sesame oil. Pour this dressing over the vegetable mixture and toss to coat.

3. Fill a shallow dish with warm water. Working with one rice paper wrapper at a time, dip it in the water for 10-15 seconds until softened.

4. Place the softened wrapper on a clean work surface. Spoon 2-3 tbsp of the vegetable filling onto the lower third of the wrapper. Fold the bottom edge over the filling, then fold in the sides and roll up tightly.

5. Place the finished spring roll seam-side down on a platter. Repeat with the remaining wrappers and filling.

6. For the dipping sauce, whisk together all the sauce ingredients in a small bowl.

7. Serve the vegetarian spring rolls immediately with the dipping sauce on the side.

For a romantic presentation, you can arrange the spring rolls in a circular pattern on a platter, garnished with extra herbs or sesame seeds. The fresh, crunchy vegetables and the sweet-savory dipping sauce make for a light and refreshing date night meal.

Enjoy these vegetarian spring rolls together with your partner for a special, intimate evening.

What is the total cooking time, including prep time?

Prep Time : _______________

Cook Time : _______________

Servings   : _______________

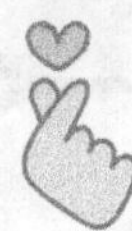

Ingredients:

- 4 pieces of beef marrow bones, about 1 lb total
- 2 tbsp olive oil
- 1 tsp coarse sea salt
- 1/2 tsp freshly ground black pepper
- 2 tbsp chopped parsley
- 1 tbsp capers, rinsed and chopped
- 1 shallot, finely minced
- Lemon wedges, for serving
- Toasted bread or crostini

Is the recipe easy to follow?

61. Roasted bone marrow

Procedure:

1. Preheat your oven to 400°F.

2. Use a sharp knife to slice the marrow bones in half lengthwise, exposing the marrow inside.

3. Arrange the bone halves cut-side up on a baking sheet. Drizzle the marrow with the olive oil and season generously with the salt and pepper.

4. Roast the bone marrow for 15-20 minutes, until the marrow is soft and starting to ooze out of the bones.

5. Remove the roasted bone marrow from the oven and sprinkle with the chopped parsley, capers, and minced shallot.

6. Serve the roasted bone marrow immediately with the lemon wedges and toasted bread or crostini on the side.

For a romantic presentation, you can arrange the roasted bone marrow halves on a wooden board or platter. Provide small spoons or forks for guests to scoop out the rich, creamy marrow.

The decadent, buttery bone marrow paired with the bright, briny garnishes makes for an indulgent and intimate date night dish. Enjoy this together with your partner, spreading the marrow on the toasted bread for a truly special meal.

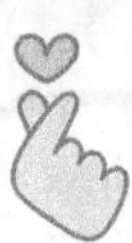

What is the total cooking time, including prep time?

Prep Time : ___________________

Cook Time : ___________________

Servings : ___________________

Ingredients:

- 4 large portobello mushroom caps, stems removed
- 2 tbsp olive oil
- Salt and pepper to taste
- 1 cup cherry tomatoes, halved
- 8 oz fresh mozzarella cheese, cut into 1/2-inch cubes
- 1/4 cup fresh basil leaves, chopped
- 2 tbsp balsamic glaze

Is the recipe easy to follow?

62. Caprese stuffed portobello mushrooms

1. Preheat your oven to 400°F. Clean the portobello mushroom caps and remove the stems. Brush the caps all over with the olive oil and season with salt and pepper.

2. Arrange the mushroom caps gill-side up on a baking sheet. Roast for 10-12 minutes until the mushrooms are tender.

3. In a medium bowl, gently toss together the cherry tomatoes, mozzarella cubes, and chopped basil.

4. Spoon the caprese filling evenly into the roasted mushroom caps, mounding it slightly on top.

5. Return the stuffed mushrooms to the oven and bake for an additional 8-10 minutes, until the cheese is melted and the filling is hot.

6. Carefully transfer the stuffed portobello mushrooms to a serving platter. Drizzle the balsamic glaze over the top.

For a romantic presentation, you can arrange the stuffed mushrooms in a circular pattern on a wooden board or platter. Garnish with extra basil leaves and serve immediately.

The juicy, savory portobello mushrooms combined with the fresh caprese-style filling make for an elegant and flavorful date night dish. Enjoy these stuffed mushrooms together with your partner for a cozy, intimate evening.

What is the total cooking time, including prep time?

Prep Time : __________________

Cook Time : __________________

Servings   : __________________

Ingredients:

- 12 large sea scallops, patted dry
- 2 tbsp unsalted butter
- 2 tbsp all-purpose flour
- 1 cup warm milk
- 1/2 cup dry white wine
- 1/4 cup heavy cream
- 2 tbsp brandy (optional)
- 1/4 cup grated Gruyère cheese
- 2 tbsp panko breadcrumbs
- 2 tbsp chopped fresh parsley
- Salt and pepper to taste

Is the recipe easy to follow?

63. Coquilles Saint-Jacques

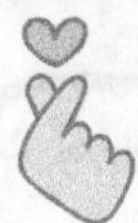

Procedure:

1. Preheat your oven to 400°F. Grease 4 individual ramekins or a small baking dish.

2. In a skillet, melt the butter over medium heat. Add the scallops and sear for 2-3 minutes per side until lightly browned. Transfer the scallops to a plate.

3. In the same skillet, whisk in the flour and cook for 1 minute. Gradually whisk in the warm milk and white wine. Bring the sauce to a simmer and cook until thickened, about 5 minutes.

4. Remove the sauce from heat and stir in the heavy cream and brandy (if using). Season with salt and pepper to taste.

5. Arrange the seared scallops in the prepared ramekins or baking dish. Pour the creamy sauce over the top, making sure to coat the scallops evenly.

6. In a small bowl, mix together the Gruyère cheese, panko breadcrumbs, and chopped parsley. Sprinkle this topping over the scallops.

7. Bake for 12-15 minutes, until the topping is golden brown and the sauce is bubbling.

8. Serve the Coquilles Saint-Jacques hot, garnished with extra parsley if desired.

For a romantic presentation, you can serve the scallops au gratin in individual ramekins or on a shared platter. The rich, creamy sauce and crispy topping make this an indulgent and elegant date night dish.

Enjoy this Coquilles Saint-Jacques together with your partner, perhaps with a glass of crisp white wine, for a truly special evening.

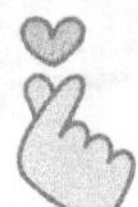

What is the total cooking time, including prep time?

Prep Time : ______________

Cook Time : ______________

Servings : ______________

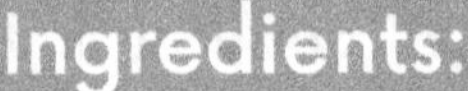 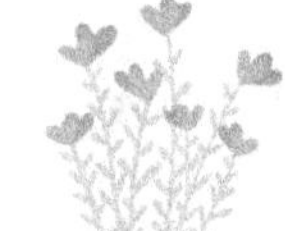

Ingredients:

- 2 medium eggplants, halved lengthwise
- 2 tbsp olive oil, plus more for drizzling
- 1 onion, finely chopped
- 3 cloves garlic, minced
- 1 lb ground lamb or beef
- 1 tsp ground cinnamon
- 1 tsp ground cumin
- 1/2 tsp crushed red pepper flakes
- 1 cup cooked rice
- 1/2 cup crumbled feta cheese
- 2 tbsp chopped fresh parsley
- Salt and pepper to taste
- Lemon wedges, for serving

Is the recipe easy to follow?

64. Stuffed eggplant

1. Preheat your oven to 375°F. Use a sharp knife to carefully slice the eggplants in half lengthwise. Scoop out the flesh, leaving about 1/4-inch of the eggplant skin intact to create boats.

2. Finely chop the scooped-out eggplant flesh. In a large skillet, heat the 2 tbsp of olive oil over medium heat. Add the chopped eggplant, onion, and garlic. Sauté for 5-7 minutes until softened.

3. Add the ground meat to the skillet and cook, breaking it up with a wooden spoon, until browned, about 5 minutes. Stir in the cinnamon, cumin, and red pepper flakes.

4. Remove the skillet from heat and stir in the cooked rice, feta, and parsley. Season the filling with salt and pepper to taste.

5. Arrange the eggplant halves in a baking dish. Spoon the filling evenly into the eggplant boats, mounding it slightly on top.

6. Drizzle the stuffed eggplants with a bit of olive oil. Bake for 25-30 minutes, until the eggplant is tender and the filling is hot.

7. Serve the stuffed eggplants warm, garnished with extra parsley if desired. Provide lemon wedges on the side.

For a romantic presentation, you can arrange the stuffed eggplant halves on a platter or wooden board. The vibrant colors and aromatic filling make this an elegant and flavorful date night dish.

Enjoy these stuffed eggplants together with your partner, perhaps with a side salad and a glass of red wine, for a cozy and intimate evening.

What is the total cooking time, including prep time?

Prep Time : ______________

Cook Time : ______________

Servings : ______________

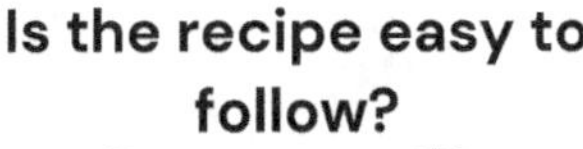
Ingredients:

- 4 boneless, skinless chicken breasts, pounded thin
- 1/4 cup all-purpose flour
- 2 tbsp olive oil
- 2 tbsp unsalted butter
- 1/2 cup dry white wine
- 1/4 cup fresh lemon juice
- 2 tbsp capers, rinsed and drained
- 2 tbsp chopped fresh parsley
- Salt and pepper to taste
- Lemon wedges, for serving

Is the recipe easy to follow?

65. Chicken piccata

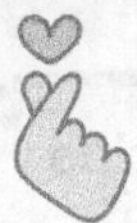
Procedure:

1. Season the pounded chicken breasts with salt and pepper. Dredge them lightly in the flour, shaking off any excess.

2. In a large skillet, heat the olive oil and 1 tbsp of the butter over medium-high heat. Working in batches if needed, add the chicken breasts and cook for 3-4 minutes per side until golden brown. Transfer the cooked chicken to a plate.

3. Add the white wine to the skillet, scraping up any browned bits from the bottom of the pan. Allow the wine to simmer for 2-3 minutes until slightly reduced.

4. Stir in the lemon juice, capers, and remaining 1 tbsp of butter. Bring the sauce to a simmer and cook for 1-2 minutes until thickened slightly.

5. Return the cooked chicken breasts to the skillet and spoon the sauce over the top. Simmer for 2-3 minutes to allow the chicken to reheat and the flavors to meld.

6. Remove from heat and sprinkle the chicken piccata with the chopped parsley.

7. Serve the chicken piccata immediately, with lemon wedges on the side.

For a romantic presentation, you can arrange the chicken breasts on a platter and spoon the lemon-caper sauce over the top. Garnish with extra parsley and lemon wedges.

The bright, tangy flavors of the piccata sauce paired with the tender, juicy chicken make this an elegant and indulgent date night dish. Enjoy it together with your partner, perhaps with a side of pasta or roasted vegetables.

What is the total cooking time, including prep time?

Prep Time : ________________

Cook Time : ________________

Servings   : ________________

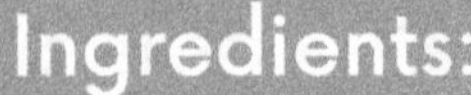

Ingredients:

- 4 cups vegetable broth, heated and kept warm
- 2 tbsp olive oil
- 1 onion, finely chopped
- 2 cloves garlic, minced
- 1 cup Arborio rice
- 1/2 cup dry white wine
- 1 cup diced butternut squash
- 1 cup sliced mushrooms
- 1/2 cup frozen peas
- 1/2 cup grated Parmesan cheese
- 2 tbsp chopped fresh parsley
- Salt and pepper to taste

Is the recipe easy to follow?

66. Vegetarian risotto

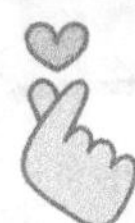

Procedure:

1. In a medium saucepan, heat the olive oil over medium heat. Add the onion and garlic and sauté for 2-3 minutes until fragrant.

2. Add the Arborio rice and stir to coat with the oil. Pour in the white wine and let it simmer, stirring frequently, until the wine is absorbed.

3. Ladle in about 1/2 cup of the warm vegetable broth and stir constantly until the liquid is absorbed. Continue this process, adding more broth 1/2 cup at a time, until the rice is tender and creamy, about 20-25 minutes total.

4. Stir in the diced butternut squash, sliced mushrooms, and frozen peas. Cook for an additional 5-7 minutes, until the vegetables are tender.

5. Remove the risotto from heat and stir in the Parmesan cheese and chopped parsley. Season with salt and pepper to taste.

6. Serve the vegetarian risotto immediately, garnished with extra parsley if desired.

For a romantic presentation, you can serve the risotto in individual bowls or on a shared platter. The vibrant colors and creamy texture make this an elegant and comforting date night dish.

Pair the risotto with a crisp white wine or a light salad for a complete romantic meal. Enjoy this vegetarian risotto together with your partner for a cozy, intimate evening.

What are the critical points in the recipe (e.g., temperature control, timing)?

What is the total cooking time, including prep time?

Prep Time   : _______________

Cook Time : _______________

Servings   : _______________

Ingredients:

- 8 oz beef tenderloin, trimmed of fat and sinew
- 2 tbsp olive oil
- 1 tbsp lemon juice
- 1 tsp Dijon mustard
- 1 tsp capers, rinsed and chopped
- 2 tbsp shaved Parmesan cheese
- 2 tbsp arugula leaves
- Salt and freshly ground black pepper

Is the recipe easy to follow?

67. Beef carpaccio

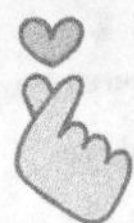

Procedure:

1. Place the beef tenderloin in the freezer for 30-60 minutes to firm up slightly, making it easier to slice.

2. In a small bowl, whisk together the olive oil, lemon juice, and Dijon mustard. Season with a pinch of salt and pepper.

3. Remove the beef from the freezer and, using a very sharp knife, slice it into paper-thin slices. Arrange the slices in a single layer on a large plate or platter.

4. Drizzle the lemon-Dijon dressing evenly over the beef carpaccio. Sprinkle with the chopped capers and shaved Parmesan.

5. Top the carpaccio with the fresh arugula leaves, arranging them attractively over the top.

6. Season the dish with additional salt and freshly ground black pepper to taste.

For a romantic presentation, you can arrange the beef carpaccio in an overlapping circular pattern on a large platter. Garnish with extra arugula, Parmesan, and a drizzle of the dressing around the edges.

The delicate, raw beef paired with the bright, tangy dressing and salty Parmesan makes for an elegant and indulgent date night appetizer. Serve this beef carpaccio with a crisp white wine or sparkling wine for a truly special evening.

Enjoy this romantic carpaccio dish together with your partner as a luxurious start to your date night.

What are the critical points in the recipe (e.g., temperature control, timing)?

What is the total cooking time, including prep time?

Prep Time : ___________________

Cook Time : ___________________

Servings   : ___________________

Ingredients:

- 1 large head green cabbage
- 1 lb ground beef or ground turkey
- 1 cup cooked rice
- 1 onion, finely chopped
- 2 cloves garlic, minced
- 1 egg, lightly beaten
- 1/4 cup chopped parsley
- 1 tsp paprika
- Salt and pepper to taste
- 1 (15 oz) can tomato sauce
- 1/4 cup brown sugar
- 2 tbsp lemon juice

Is the recipe easy to follow?

68. Stuffed cabbage rolls

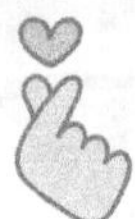

Procedure:

1. Bring a large pot of water to a boil. Using a paring knife, carefully core the cabbage and place it in the boiling water. Cook for 2-3 minutes until the outer leaves are softened. Remove the cabbage and let cool slightly.

2. Carefully peel off the softened cabbage leaves, keeping them intact. You should have about 12-14 leaves.

3. In a large bowl, combine the ground meat, cooked rice, onion, garlic, egg, parsley, paprika, salt, and pepper. Mix well until fully incorporated.

4. Place about 2-3 tablespoons of the meat mixture onto the center of each cabbage leaf. Fold the sides of the leaf over the filling, then roll up tightly.

5. Arrange the stuffed cabbage rolls seam-side down in a baking dish.

6. In a small bowl, whisk together the tomato sauce, brown sugar, and lemon juice. Pour this sauce over the stuffed cabbage rolls.

7. Cover the baking dish with foil and bake at 350°F for 45-60 minutes, until the cabbage is tender and the filling is cooked through.

8. Serve the stuffed cabbage rolls warm, spooning the sauce over the top.

For a romantic presentation, you can arrange the stuffed cabbage rolls in a circular pattern on a platter. Garnish with extra parsley or lemon wedges.

The savory, hearty filling paired with the tangy tomato sauce makes these stuffed cabbage rolls an elegant and comforting date night dish. Enjoy them together with your partner, perhaps with a side of mashed potatoes or a fresh salad.

What is the total cooking time, including prep time?

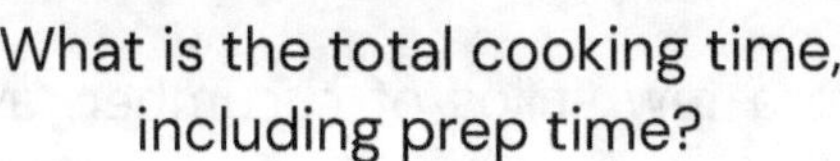

Prep Time : _________________

Cook Time : _________________

Servings : _________________

Ingredients:

- 12 fresh sardines, cleaned and butterflied
- 2 tbsp olive oil
- 1 lemon, cut into wedges
- Salt and pepper to taste

Is the recipe easy to follow?

69. Grilled sardines

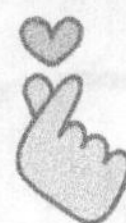

Procedure:

1. Preheat grill or grill pan to medium-high heat.

2. Rinse the sardines under cold water and pat them dry with paper towels. Brush both sides of the sardines with olive oil and season generously with salt and pepper.

3. Place the sardines skin-side down on the hot grill. Grill for 2-3 minutes per side, until the skin is crispy and the flesh is opaque throughout.

4. Transfer the grilled sardines to a serving platter. Serve immediately with lemon wedges on the side.

Tips:
- Look for fresh, high-quality sardines. Avoid any that smell fishy.
- You can also marinate the sardines in olive oil, lemon juice, garlic, and herbs before grilling.
- Serve the grilled sardines with crusty bread, a fresh salad, or roasted potatoes.

Enjoy your grilled sardines!

What is the total cooking time, including prep time?

Prep Time : ___________________

Cook Time : ___________________

Servings : ___________________

Ingredients:

- 2 cups sushi rice, cooked and cooled
- 4-6 sheets nori (seaweed sheets)
- 1 cucumber, peeled, seeded and cut into thin strips
- 1 avocado, sliced
- 1 carrot, peeled and cut into thin strips
- 1 red bell pepper, seeded and cut into thin strips
- 1 cup shredded purple cabbage
- Toasted sesame seeds for garnish
- Soy sauce, wasabi and pickled ginger for serving

Is the recipe easy to follow?

70. Vegetarian sushi rolls

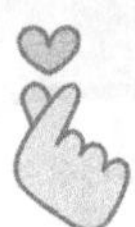

Procedure:

1. Lay a sheet of nori shiny-side down on a bamboo sushi mat. Spread about 1/2 cup of the sushi rice evenly over the nori, leaving a 1-inch border at the top.

2. Arrange a few strips of cucumber, avocado, carrot, bell pepper and cabbage in a line across the center of the rice.

3. Starting from the bottom, use the sushi mat to tightly roll the nori around the fillings. Moisten the top edge with a bit of water to seal the roll.

4. Repeat with the remaining nori sheets and fillings.

5. Slice each roll into 6-8 pieces using a very sharp knife. Wet the knife between cuts to prevent sticking.

6. Arrange the sushi rolls on a platter and sprinkle with toasted sesame seeds.

7. Serve the vegetarian sushi rolls immediately with soy sauce, wasabi and pickled ginger on the side.

Enjoy your homemade vegetarian sushi rolls!

What is the total cooking time, including prep time?

Prep Time : _______________

Cook Time : _______________

Servings   : _______________

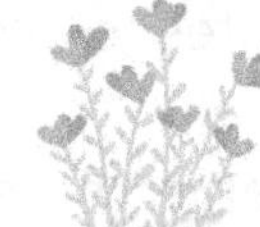

Ingredients:

- 2 Cornish game hens, rinsed and patted dry
- 2 tbsp olive oil
- 2 tsp dried thyme
- 1 tsp garlic powder
- 1 tsp salt
- 1/2 tsp black pepper
- 1 lemon, cut into wedges

Is the recipe easy to follow?

71. Roasted Cornish game hen

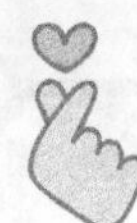

Procedure:

1. Preheat your oven to 400°F (200°C).

2. In a small bowl, mix together the olive oil, thyme, garlic powder, salt, and black pepper.

3. Place the Cornish game hens on a rimmed baking sheet. Rub the seasoning mixture all over the outside of the hens, making sure to get it into all the nooks and crannies.

4. Roast the hens in the preheated oven for 45-55 minutes, or until the internal temperature reaches 165°F (75°C) when measured in the thickest part of the thigh.

5. Remove the hens from the oven and let them rest for 5-10 minutes before serving.

6. Serve the roasted Cornish game hens warm, with the lemon wedges on the side. The lemon can be squeezed over the top of the hens just before eating.

Tips:
- You can stuff the cavity of the hens with herbs, garlic, or lemon slices for extra flavor.
- Baste the hens with the pan juices a few times during roasting for extra crispy skin.
- Serve the roasted Cornish game hens with roasted potatoes, a fresh salad, or your favorite vegetable side dish.

Enjoy your delicious roasted Cornish game hens! .

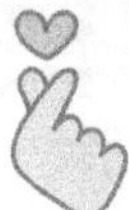

What is the total cooking time, including prep time?

Prep Time : _______________

Cook Time : _______________

Servings   : _______________

Ingredients:

- 12-15 peppadew peppers, stems removed and halved
- 4 oz cream cheese, softened
- 1/4 cup crumbled feta cheese
- 2 tbsp chopped fresh parsley
- 1 tbsp chopped fresh basil
- 1 garlic clove, minced
- Salt and pepper to taste

Is the recipe easy to follow?

72. Stuffed peppadew peppers

1. In a medium bowl, mix together the cream cheese, feta cheese, parsley, basil, garlic, salt, and pepper until well combined.

2. Carefully spoon or pipe the cheese mixture into the hollowed-out peppadew pepper halves, filling them evenly.

3. Arrange the stuffed peppers on a serving platter or baking sheet.

4. Refrigerate the stuffed peppers for at least 30 minutes to allow the filling to firm up.

5. Serve the stuffed peppadew peppers chilled or at room temperature as an appetizer.

Tips:
- Peppadew peppers are sweet, tangy, and slightly spicy. You can find them jarred or fresh in the produce section of many grocery stores.
- For a spicier version, add a pinch of crushed red pepper flakes to the cheese filling.
- Try using different herbs or cheese varieties to change up the flavor profile.
- These stuffed peppers can be made ahead of time and refrigerated until ready to serve.

Enjoy these flavorful and easy-to-make stuffed peppadew peppers!

What are the critical points in the recipe (e.g., temperature control, timing)?

What is the total cooking time, including prep time?

Prep Time : ______________

Cook Time : ______________

Servings   : ______________

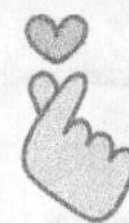

Ingredients:

- 2 lbs fresh mussels, scrubbed and debearded
- 2 tbsp olive oil
- 3 garlic cloves, minced
- 1 shallot, finely chopped
- 1 cup dry white wine
- 1 cup heavy cream
- 2 tbsp unsalted butter
- 2 tbsp chopped fresh parsley
- Salt and pepper to taste
- Crusty bread, for serving

Is the recipe easy to follow?

73. Mussels in white wine sauce

Procedure:

1. Rinse the mussels under cold running water, scrubbing off any dirt or debris. Remove the beards (the fibrous strings) by pulling them off with your fingers. Discard any mussels that are cracked or won't close when tapped.

2. In a large pot or Dutch oven, heat the olive oil over medium heat. Add the garlic and shallot and cook for 1-2 minutes, until fragrant.

3. Pour in the white wine and bring to a simmer. Add the mussels, cover the pot, and cook for 5-7 minutes, stirring occasionally, until the mussels have opened up.

4. Remove the lid and stir in the heavy cream and butter. Cook for an additional 2-3 minutes, until the sauce has thickened slightly.

5. Stir in the chopped parsley and season with salt and pepper to taste.

6. Serve the mussels immediately in shallow bowls, with the sauce spooned over the top. Provide crusty bread for dipping in the delicious sauce.

Tips:
- Pair the mussels with a crisp, dry white wine for the ultimate romantic date night meal.
- Dim the lights, light some candles, and enjoy this elegant and indulgent seafood dish together.
- For an extra special touch, garnish with lemon wedges and additional parsley.

Enjoy your romantic mussels in white wine sauce!

What is the total cooking time, including prep time?

Prep Time : _______________

Cook Time : _______________

Servings : _______________

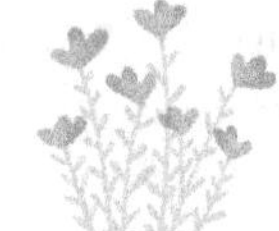

Ingredients:

- 12-15 squash blossoms, stems and pistils removed
- 4 oz ricotta cheese
- 2 tbsp grated Parmesan cheese
- 1 tbsp chopped fresh basil
- 1 garlic clove, minced
- Salt and pepper to taste
- 1/2 cup all-purpose flour
- 1/2 cup sparkling water or soda water
- Vegetable oil for frying

Is the recipe easy to follow?

74. Stuffed squash blossoms

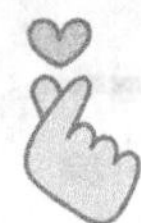

Procedure:

1. In a small bowl, mix together the ricotta, Parmesan, basil, garlic, salt, and pepper until well combined.

2. Carefully stuff each squash blossom with about 1-2 tsp of the ricotta mixture, gently twisting the petals to enclose the filling.

3. In a shallow bowl, whisk together the flour and sparkling water to make a light batter.

4. In a large skillet or Dutch oven, heat about 2-3 inches of vegetable oil to 350°F.

5. Working in batches, dip the stuffed squash blossoms into the batter, allowing any excess to drip off.

6. Carefully lower the battered blossoms into the hot oil and fry for 2-3 minutes per side, until golden brown.

7. Transfer the fried stuffed squash blossoms to a paper towel-lined plate to drain.

8. Serve the warm, crispy stuffed squash blossoms immediately, garnished with additional basil if desired.

Tips:
- Look for fresh, unblemished squash blossoms at your local farmers market or specialty grocery store.
- You can also use a mixture of ricotta and goat cheese for the filling.
- For a crispier batter, use club soda or sparkling water instead of regular water.
- Serve the stuffed squash blossoms as an appetizer or light main course.

Enjoy these delicate and flavorful stuffed squash blossoms!

What is the total cooking time, including prep time?

Prep Time : _______________

Cook Time : _______________

Servings : _______________

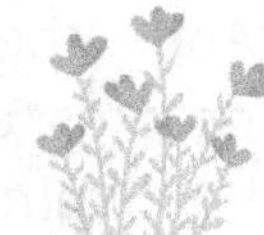

Ingredients:

- 8 veal scaloppine, pounded thin
- 8 thin slices prosciutto
- 8 fresh sage leaves
- 2 tbsp olive oil
- 1/2 cup dry white wine
- 2 tbsp unsalted butter
- Salt and pepper to taste

Is the recipe easy to follow?

75. Veal saltimbocca

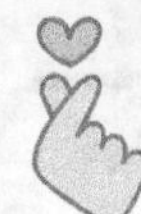

Procedure:

1. Season the veal scaloppine with salt and pepper on both sides.

2. Place a slice of prosciutto and a sage leaf on top of each veal scaloppine.

3. In a large skillet, heat the olive oil over medium-high heat.

4. Carefully add the veal scaloppine to the pan, prosciutto-side down. Cook for 2-3 minutes until the prosciutto is crispy.

5. Flip the veal and cook for an additional 2-3 minutes, until the veal is cooked through but still tender.

6. Transfer the veal saltimbocca to a plate and cover to keep warm.

7. Add the white wine to the skillet and use a wooden spoon to scrape up any browned bits from the bottom of the pan.

8. Allow the wine to simmer and reduce by half, about 2-3 minutes.

9. Remove the pan from heat and stir in the butter until melted and the sauce is smooth.

10. Serve the veal saltimbocca immediately, drizzled with the white wine sauce.

Tips:
- Use high-quality prosciutto and fresh sage for the best flavor.
- Pound the veal scaloppine thin to ensure even cooking.
- Serve the veal saltimbocca with roasted potatoes or a fresh salad for a complete meal.

Enjoy this classic Italian dish of tender veal wrapped in prosciutto and sage!

What is the total cooking time, including prep time?

Prep Time : ________________

Cook Time : ________________

Servings : ________________

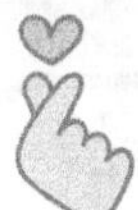

Ingredients:

- 8 cups vegetable broth
- 3 whole star anise
- 3 whole cloves
- 1 cinnamon stick
- 1 tbsp coriander seeds
- 1 tbsp fennel seeds
- 1 inch piece fresh ginger, peeled and sliced
- 8 oz rice noodles
- 1 cup thinly sliced shiitake mushrooms
- 1 cup thinly sliced oyster mushrooms
- 1 cup thinly sliced carrots
- 1 cup thinly sliced bok choy
- 2 green onions, thinly sliced
- 1/4 cup fresh cilantro leaves
- 2 tbsp hoisin sauce
- 2 tbsp sriracha or other hot sauce (optional)
- Lime wedges for serving

Is the recipe easy to follow?

76. Vegetarian pho

Procedure:

1. In a large pot, combine the vegetable broth, star anise, cloves, cinnamon stick, coriander seeds, fennel seeds, and ginger. Bring to a boil, then reduce heat and simmer for 20 minutes.

2. Strain the broth through a fine mesh sieve, discarding the solids. Return the broth to the pot and keep warm.

3. Cook the rice noodles according to package instructions. Drain and set aside.

4. Add the shiitake mushrooms, oyster mushrooms, carrots, and bok choy to the warm broth. Simmer for 5-7 minutes until the vegetables are tender.

5. To serve, divide the cooked noodles among 4 bowls. Ladle the hot broth and vegetables over the noodles. Top each bowl with sliced green onions and cilantro leaves.

6. Provide hoisin sauce and sriracha on the side for guests to customize their pho to their desired level of sweetness and spice.

7. Serve the vegetarian pho immediately, with lime wedges on the side.

Tips:
- For a romantic date night, dim the lights, light some candles, and play soft music in the background.
- Provide crusty bread or baguettes for dipping in the flavorful broth.
- Encourage your date to slurp the noodles - it's part of the experience!

Enjoy this fragrant and comforting vegetarian pho together on your date night.

What is the total cooking time,
including prep time?

Prep Time : ________________

Cook Time : ________________

Servings   : ________________

Ingredients:

- 1 lb beef tenderloin or sirloin, trimmed
- 2 tbsp soy sauce
- 1 tbsp rice vinegar
- 1 tbsp sesame oil
- 1 tsp grated ginger
- 1 garlic clove, minced
- 1 tsp sesame seeds
- 2 green onions, thinly sliced
- Microgreens or sprouts for garnish

Dipping Sauce:
- 2 tbsp soy sauce
- 1 tbsp rice vinegar
- 1 tsp sesame oil
- 1 tsp honey
- 1 tsp grated ginger

Is the recipe easy to follow?

77. Beef tataki

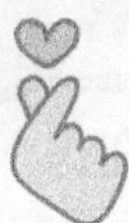

Procedure:

1. In a shallow dish, combine the soy sauce, rice vinegar, sesame oil, ginger, and garlic. Add the beef and turn to coat evenly. Cover and refrigerate for 30 minutes to 1 hour.

2. In a small bowl, whisk together the dipping sauce ingredients and set aside.

3. Heat a large skillet or grill pan over high heat. Sear the beef on all sides until a nice crust forms, about 2-3 minutes per side. The center should still be rare.

4. Transfer the beef to a cutting board and let rest for 5-10 minutes. Slice the beef into thin, diagonal slices.

5. Arrange the sliced beef tataki on a serving platter. Sprinkle with sesame seeds and green onions.

6. Serve the beef tataki immediately, with the dipping sauce on the side. Garnish with microgreens or sprouts.

Tips for a Romantic Date Night:
- Dim the lights and light some candles to set the mood.
- Pair the beef tataki with a crisp white wine or sake.
- Encourage your date to dip the beef in the sauce and savor the flavors together.
- Slow down and enjoy the experience - this dish is meant to be savored.
- Provide chopsticks for an authentic Japanese dining experience.

Enjoy your romantic beef tataki date night!

What is the total cooking time, including prep time?

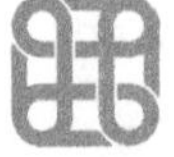 Prep Time : _______________

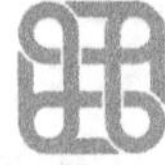 Cook Time : _______________

Servings : _______________

Ingredients:

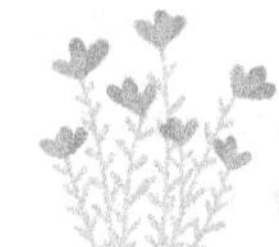

- 4 large sweet onions
- 1 cup cooked rice
- 1/2 cup crumbled feta cheese
- 1/4 cup chopped fresh parsley
- 2 tbsp olive oil, plus more for drizzling
- 2 garlic cloves, minced
- Salt and pepper to taste
- Balsamic glaze for drizzling (optional)

Is the recipe easy to follow?

78. Stuffed onions

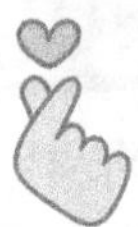

Procedure:

1. Preheat your oven to 375°F (190°C).

2. Slice the tops and bottoms off the onions, then carefully scoop out the centers, leaving a 1/2-inch thick shell. Finely chop the scooped-out onion centers.

3. In a medium bowl, combine the chopped onion centers, cooked rice, feta cheese, parsley, 2 tbsp olive oil, and garlic. Season with salt and pepper.

4. Stuff the onion shells evenly with the rice mixture, packing it in gently.

5. Place the stuffed onions in a baking dish and drizzle with a bit of olive oil.

6. Bake for 45-55 minutes, or until the onions are tender and the filling is hot and lightly browned.

7. Remove the stuffed onions from the oven and let them cool for a few minutes.

8. Serve the warm stuffed onions drizzled with balsamic glaze, if desired.

Tips for a Romantic Date Night:
- Dim the lights and light some candles to create a cozy, intimate atmosphere.
- Pair the stuffed onions with a crisp white wine or a light red.
- Encourage your date to share the stuffed onions, taking turns dipping and savoring the flavors.
- Slow down and enjoy the experience - this dish is meant to be shared and savored.
- Provide small plates and forks to make it easy to share the stuffed onions.

Enjoy your romantic stuffed onions date night!

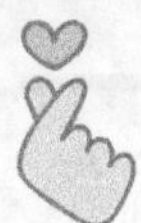

What is the total cooking time, including prep time?

Prep Time : _______________

Cook Time : _______________

Servings : _______________

Ingredients:

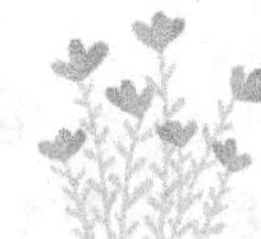

- 1 lb fresh calamari, cleaned and cut into rings
- 2 tbsp olive oil
- 2 tbsp lemon juice
- 2 garlic cloves, minced
- 1 tsp dried oregano
- Salt and pepper to taste
- Lemon wedges for serving

Dipping Sauce:
- 1/4 cup olive oil
- 2 tbsp lemon juice
- 2 tbsp chopped fresh parsley
- 1 garlic clove, minced
- 1/4 tsp red pepper flakes
- Salt and pepper to taste

Is the recipe easy to follow?

79. Grilled calamari

1. In a large bowl, combine the calamari rings, 2 tbsp olive oil, lemon juice, garlic, and oregano. Toss to coat the calamari evenly. Season with salt and pepper.

2. Prepare your grill for high, direct heat. If using a grill basket, lightly oil it to prevent sticking.

3. Grill the calamari for 2-3 minutes per side, until lightly charred and cooked through. Be careful not to overcook.

4. While the calamari is grilling, make the dipping sauce. In a small bowl, whisk together the 1/4 cup olive oil, lemon juice, parsley, garlic, red pepper flakes, salt, and pepper.

5. Transfer the grilled calamari to a serving platter. Serve immediately with the dipping sauce and lemon wedges on the side.

Tips for a Romantic Date Night:

- Dim the lights and light some candles to create a cozy, intimate atmosphere.

- Pair the grilled calamari with a crisp white wine or a light, chilled rosé.

- Encourage your date to dip the calamari in the sauce and savor the flavors together.

- Slow down and enjoy the experience - this dish is meant to be shared and savored.

- Provide small plates and forks to make it easy to share the calamari.

Enjoy your romantic grilled calamari date night!

What is the total cooking time, including prep time?

Prep Time   : _______________

Cook Time : _______________

Servings   : _______________

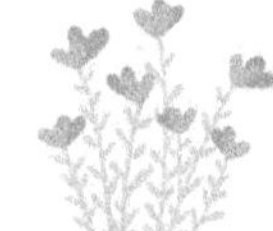

Ingredients:

- 8 oz rice vermicelli noodles
- 1 cup shredded cabbage
- 1 cup shredded carrots
- 1 cup thinly sliced cucumber
- 1/2 cup thinly sliced red bell pepper
- 1/4 cup chopped fresh mint
- 1/4 cup chopped fresh cilantro
- 12 round rice paper wrappers
- Hoisin sauce and sriracha for serving

For the Dipping Sauce:
- 1/4 cup hoisin sauce
- 2 tbsp rice vinegar
- 1 tbsp soy sauce
- 1 tsp sesame oil
- 1 garlic clove, minced
- 1 tsp grated ginger

Is the recipe easy to follow?

80. Vegetarian spring rolls

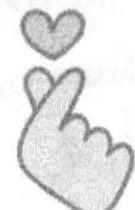

Procedure:

1. Cook the rice vermicelli noodles according to package instructions. Drain and rinse under cold water. Set aside.

2. In a large bowl, combine the cooked noodles, cabbage, carrots, cucumber, bell pepper, mint, and cilantro. Toss gently to mix.

3. Fill a shallow dish with warm water. Dip one rice paper wrapper into the water for 10-15 seconds until softened. Transfer to a clean work surface.

4. Place a few tablespoons of the vegetable filling in the center of the wrapper. Fold the bottom edge over the filling, then fold in the sides and roll up tightly.

5. Repeat with the remaining wrappers and filling.

6. In a small bowl, whisk together all the dipping sauce ingredients.

7. Arrange the spring rolls on a serving platter. Serve immediately with the dipping sauce on the side.

Tips for a Romantic Date Night:
- Dim the lights and light some candles to create a cozy, intimate atmosphere.
- Pair the spring rolls with a crisp white wine or a refreshing cocktail.
- Encourage your date to dip the spring rolls in the sauce and share the experience.
- Slow down and enjoy the process of assembling the spring rolls together.
- Provide small plates and chopsticks for an authentic dining experience.

Enjoy your romantic vegetarian spring rolls date night!

Prep Time : ________________

Cook Time : ________________

Servings   : ________________

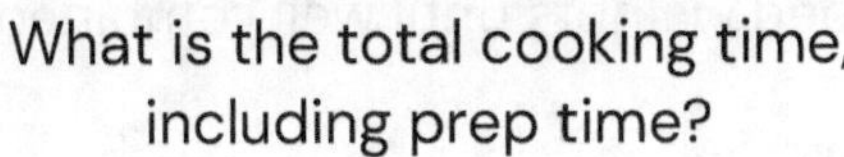

Ingredients:

- 2 whole pheasants, rinsed and patted dry
- 4 tbsp unsalted butter, softened
- 2 tsp dried thyme
- 1 tsp garlic powder
- 1 tsp salt
- 1/2 tsp black pepper
- 1 lemon, cut into wedges
- 1 cup dry white wine

Is the recipe easy to follow?

81. Roasted pheasant

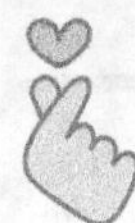

Procedure:

1. Preheat your oven to 400°F (200°C).

2. In a small bowl, mix together the softened butter, thyme, garlic powder, salt, and black pepper.

3. Gently loosen the skin of the pheasants and spread the seasoned butter mixture under the skin, covering the breasts and legs.

4. Place the pheasants in a roasting pan and pour the white wine around the birds.

5. Roast the pheasants in the preheated oven for 60-75 minutes, basting with the pan juices every 15 minutes, until the internal temperature reaches 165°F (75°C) when measured in the thickest part of the thigh.

6. Remove the pheasants from the oven and let them rest for 10-15 minutes before carving.

7. Carve the pheasants and arrange the pieces on a serving platter. Drizzle with the pan juices and serve with the lemon wedges.

Tips for a Romantic Date Night:
- Dim the lights and light some candles to create a cozy, intimate atmosphere.
- Pair the roasted pheasant with a full-bodied red wine or a crisp white wine.
- Serve the pheasant with a side of roasted potatoes or a fresh salad.
- Encourage your date to savor the tender, flavorful meat and share the experience.
- Provide small plates and utensils to make it easy to share the pheasant.

Enjoy your romantic roasted pheasant date night!

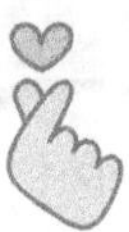

What is the total cooking time, including prep time?

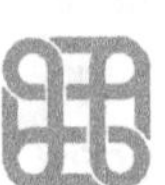 Prep Time : _______________

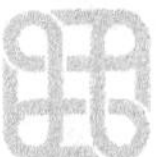 Cook Time : _______________

Servings : _______________

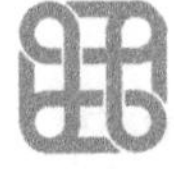

Ingredients:
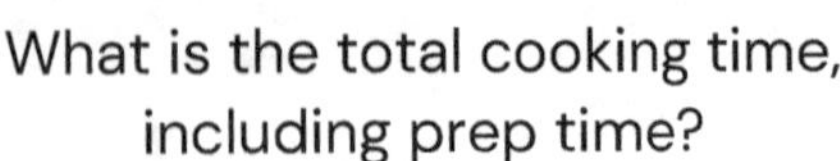

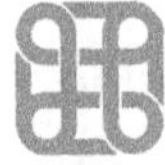

- 12 Medjool dates, pitted
- 2 oz goat cheese, softened
- 2 tbsp chopped toasted walnuts
- 12 slices of bacon, cut in half crosswise

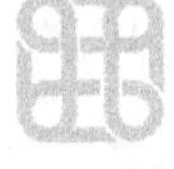

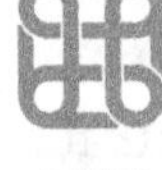

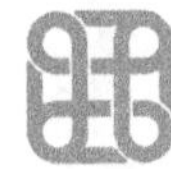

Is the recipe easy to follow?

82. Stuffed dates wrapped in bacon

1. Preheat your oven to 400°F (200°C). Line a baking sheet with parchment paper.

2. In a small bowl, mix together the goat cheese and chopped walnuts until well combined.

3. Carefully slice each date lengthwise, leaving one side intact, to create a pocket. Spoon about 1 tsp of the goat cheese mixture into the pocket of each date.

4. Wrap each stuffed date with a half slice of bacon, securing it with a toothpick.

5. Arrange the bacon-wrapped dates on the prepared baking sheet.

6. Bake for 18-22 minutes, or until the bacon is crispy.

7. Remove the toothpicks and transfer the stuffed dates to a serving platter.

Tips for a Romantic Date Night:
- Dim the lights and light some candles to create a cozy, intimate atmosphere.
- Pair the stuffed dates with a glass of sparkling wine or a light cocktail.
- Encourage your date to share the dates, taking turns enjoying the sweet and savory flavors.
- Slow down and savor the experience - these bites are meant to be enjoyed slowly.
- Provide small plates or napkins to make it easy to share the stuffed dates.

Enjoy your romantic stuffed dates wrapped in bacon date night!

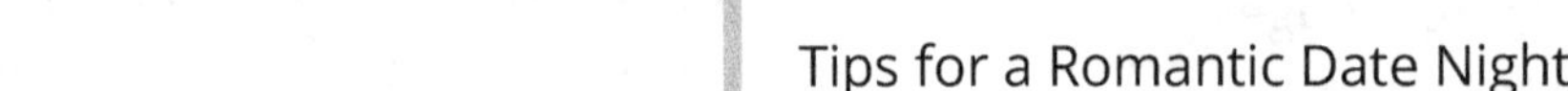

What is the total cooking time, including prep time?

Prep Time : _________________

Cook Time : _________________

Servings   : _________________

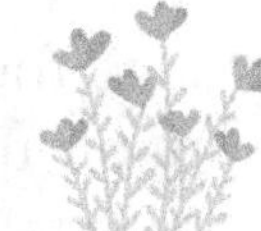

Ingredients:

- 12 large sea scallops, patted dry
- 6 slices of thick-cut bacon, cut in half crosswise
- 2 tbsp unsalted butter
- 1 tbsp olive oil
- 2 tbsp dry white wine
- 1 tbsp lemon juice
- 2 tbsp chopped fresh parsley
- Salt and pepper to taste

Is the recipe easy to follow?

83. Scallops with bacon

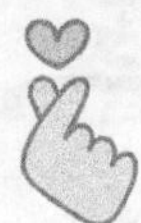

Procedure:

1. Wrap each scallop with a half slice of bacon, securing it with a toothpick.

2. In a large skillet, heat the butter and olive oil over medium-high heat.

3. Add the bacon-wrapped scallops to the skillet and cook for 2-3 minutes per side, or until the bacon is crispy and the scallops are opaque and cooked through.

4. Transfer the scallops to a plate and cover to keep warm.

5. Add the white wine and lemon juice to the skillet, scraping up any browned bits from the bottom of the pan.

6. Allow the sauce to simmer for 1-2 minutes, until slightly reduced.

7. Remove the toothpicks from the scallops and arrange them on a serving platter.

8. Drizzle the white wine sauce over the scallops and sprinkle with the chopped parsley.

9. Season with salt and pepper to taste.

Tips for a Romantic Date Night:
- Dim the lights and light some candles to create a cozy, intimate atmosphere.
- Pair the scallops with a crisp white wine or a light, chilled rosé.
- Encourage your date to share the scallops, taking turns enjoying the sweet and savory flavors.
- Slow down and savor the experience - these scallops are meant to be enjoyed slowly.
- Provide small plates and forks to make it easy to share the scallops.

What is the total cooking time, including prep time?

Prep Time : _________________

Cook Time : _________________

Servings : _________________

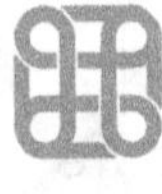
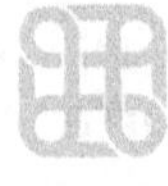
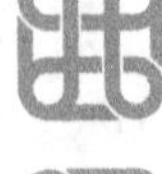
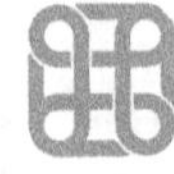

Ingredients:

- 4 large portobello mushroom caps, stems removed and chopped
- 2 tbsp olive oil, plus more for drizzling
- 1 shallot, finely chopped
- 2 garlic cloves, minced
- 1/2 cup cooked quinoa
- 1/2 cup crumbled feta cheese
- 2 tbsp chopped fresh basil
- Salt and pepper to taste
- Balsamic glaze for drizzling (optional)

Is the recipe easy to follow?

84. Stuffed portobello mushrooms

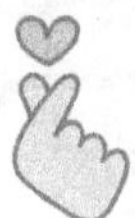

Procedure:

1. Preheat your oven to 400°F (200°C). Line a baking sheet with parchment paper.

2. In a skillet, heat the 2 tbsp of olive oil over medium heat. Add the chopped mushroom stems, shallot, and garlic. Sauté for 5-7 minutes, until the mushrooms are tender and the shallot is translucent.

3. Remove the skillet from heat and stir in the cooked quinoa, feta cheese, and chopped basil. Season with salt and pepper.

4. Arrange the portobello mushroom caps, gill-side up, on the prepared baking sheet. Spoon the quinoa-feta filling evenly into the mushroom caps.

5. Drizzle the stuffed mushrooms lightly with olive oil.

6. Bake for 15-20 minutes, or until the mushrooms are tender and the filling is hot and lightly browned.

7. Remove the stuffed portobello mushrooms from the oven and drizzle with balsamic glaze, if desired.

8. Serve the warm stuffed mushrooms immediately, garnished with additional fresh basil if desired.

Tips for a Romantic Date Night:
- Dim the lights and light some candles to create a cozy, intimate atmosphere.
- Pair the stuffed mushrooms with a crisp white wine or a light, chilled rosé.
- Encourage your date to share the stuffed mushrooms, taking turns enjoying the flavors.
- Slow down and savor the experience - these mushrooms are meant to be enjoyed slowly.
- Provide small plates and forks to make it easy to share the stuffed mushrooms.

What is the total cooking time, including prep time?

Prep Time : ___________

Cook Time : ___________

Servings : ___________

Ingredients:

- 2 whole duck breasts, skin-on
- Salt and pepper
- 1/4 cup orange juice
- 2 tbsp honey
- 2 tbsp Dijon mustard
- 1 tbsp balsamic vinegar
- 1 tbsp orange zest
- 2 tbsp unsalted butter
- 1 shallot, minced
- 1 garlic clove, minced
- 1/2 cup dry white wine
- 1 cup chicken or duck stock
- 2 tbsp orange marmalade
- Chopped parsley for garnish

Is the recipe easy to follow?

85. Duck à l'orange

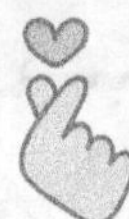

Procedure:

1. Pat the duck breasts dry and season generously with salt and pepper.

2. In a small bowl, whisk together the orange juice, honey, Dijon mustard, balsamic vinegar, and orange zest. Set aside.

3. In a large, oven-safe skillet, cook the duck breasts skin-side down over medium heat for 8-10 minutes, until the skin is crispy. Flip and cook for an additional 5-7 minutes for medium-rare. Transfer the duck to a cutting board and let rest.

4. Drain all but 2 tbsp of the duck fat from the skillet. Add the butter, shallot, and garlic. Cook for 2-3 minutes until fragrant.

5. Deglaze the pan with the white wine, scraping up any browned bits. Simmer for 2-3 minutes to reduce slightly.

6. Add the stock, orange marmalade, and the reserved orange juice mixture. Bring to a simmer and cook for 5-7 minutes, until the sauce has thickened slightly.

7. Slice the duck breasts and arrange on a serving platter. Drizzle the orange sauce over the top.

8. Garnish with chopped parsley and serve immediately.

Tips for a Romantic Date Night:
- Dim the lights and light some candles to create a cozy, intimate atmosphere.
- Pair the duck à l'orange with a full-bodied red wine or a crisp white wine.
- Serve the duck with roasted potatoes or a fresh salad for a complete meal.
- Encourage your date to savor the rich, flavorful duck and share the experience.
- Provide small plates and utensils to make it easy to share the dish.

What is the total cooking time, including prep time?

Prep Time : _______________

Cook Time : _______________

Servings : _______________

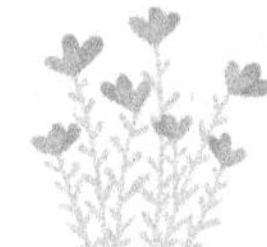

Ingredients:

- 8 oz rice noodles
- 2 tbsp vegetable oil
- 2 cloves garlic, minced
- 1 cup diced firm tofu
- 1 cup shredded cabbage or bean sprouts
- 2 eggs, lightly beaten
- 2 tbsp tamarind paste
- 2 tbsp fish sauce (use soy sauce for vegan)
- 1 tbsp brown sugar
- 1 lime, cut into wedges
- 2 tbsp chopped roasted peanuts
- 2 tbsp chopped cilantro

Is the recipe easy to follow?

86. Vegetarian pad thai

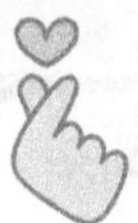

Procedure:

1. Soak the rice noodles in hot water for 15-20 minutes until softened. Drain and set aside.

2. Heat the oil in a large skillet or wok over medium-high heat. Add the garlic and sauté for 1 minute until fragrant.

3. Add the tofu and stir-fry for 2-3 minutes until lightly browned.

4. Push the tofu to the side and pour in the beaten eggs. Scramble the eggs for 1-2 minutes.

5. Add the softened noodles, cabbage/bean sprouts, tamarind paste, fish sauce (or soy sauce), and brown sugar. Toss everything together and cook for 2-3 minutes until the noodles are heated through.

6. Remove from heat and squeeze the lime juice over the top. Garnish with chopped peanuts and cilantro.

7. Serve immediately while hot. Enjoy your vegetarian pad thai!

What is the total cooking time, including prep time?

Prep Time : ________________

Cook Time : ________________

Servings   : ________________

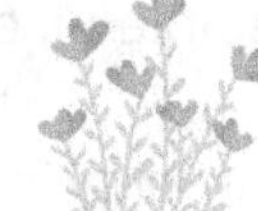

Ingredients:

- 1 lb beef tenderloin, thinly sliced into 1/4-inch strips
- 8 oz scallions, cut into 3-inch pieces
- 2 tbsp soy sauce
- 2 tbsp mirin
- 1 tbsp brown sugar
- 1 tsp sesame oil
- 1 tsp grated ginger
- 1 clove garlic, minced
- Toasted sesame seeds for garnish

Is the recipe easy to follow?

87. Beef negimaki

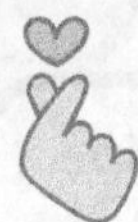

Procedure:

1. In a shallow bowl, whisk together the soy sauce, mirin, brown sugar, sesame oil, ginger, and garlic. Add the beef strips and toss to coat. Cover and marinate in the refrigerator for 30 minutes.

2. Preheat your oven to 400°F. Line a baking sheet with parchment paper.

3. Remove the beef from the marinade, reserving the marinade. Lay a piece of scallion on the end of each beef strip, then tightly roll up the beef around the scallion.

4. Arrange the beef negimaki rolls seam-side down on the prepared baking sheet.

5. Bake for 12-15 minutes, until the beef is cooked through.

6. Meanwhile, pour the reserved marinade into a small saucepan. Bring to a simmer over medium heat and cook for 2-3 minutes to thicken slightly.

7. Remove the beef negimaki from the oven. Drizzle the warm marinade sauce over the top.

8. Sprinkle the negimaki with toasted sesame seeds before serving.

For a romantic presentation, you can arrange the beef negimaki rolls on a wooden board or platter. The vibrant green scallions and the glossy, caramelized sauce make this an elegant and visually appealing date night dish.

The tender, flavorful beef wrapped around the crisp scallions creates a delightful contrast in textures and tastes. Serve the beef negimaki warm, perhaps with a side of steamed rice or a fresh salad, for a cozy and intimate date night meal.

What are the critical points in the recipe (e.g., temperature control, timing)?

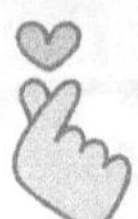

What is the total cooking time, including prep time?

Prep Time   : _______________

Cook Time : _______________

Servings   : _______________

Ingredients:

- 12 fresh zucchini flowers, stems and pistils removed
- 4 oz ricotta cheese
- 2 tbsp grated Parmesan cheese
- 1 tbsp chopped fresh basil
- 1 tsp lemon zest
- Salt and pepper to taste
- 1/4 cup all-purpose flour
- 1/4 cup sparkling water
- Vegetable oil for frying
- Lemon wedges for serving

Is the recipe easy to follow?

88. Stuffed zucchini flowers

1. In a small bowl, mix together the ricotta, Parmesan, basil, and lemon zest. Season with a pinch of salt and pepper.

2. Carefully stuff each zucchini flower with about 1-2 tbsp of the ricotta mixture, gently twisting the petals to enclose the filling.

3. In a shallow bowl, whisk together the flour and sparkling water to make a light batter.

4. In a large skillet, heat about 1/2 inch of vegetable oil over medium-high heat.

5. Working in batches, dip the stuffed zucchini flowers into the batter, allowing any excess to drip off. Carefully lower them into the hot oil.

6. Fry the stuffed flowers for 2-3 minutes per side, until golden brown and crispy. Transfer to a paper towel-lined plate.

7. Serve the warm, crispy stuffed zucchini flowers immediately, garnished with lemon wedges on the side.

For a romantic presentation, you can arrange the stuffed flowers on a platter or wooden board. The vibrant colors and delicate texture make this an elegant and indulgent date night appetizer.

The creamy ricotta filling paired with the crispy, golden batter creates a delicious contrast in flavors and textures. Enjoy these stuffed zucchini flowers together with your partner, perhaps with a glass of chilled white wine, for a truly special evening.

What is the total cooking time, including prep time?

Prep Time : _______________

Cook Time : _______________

Servings : _______________

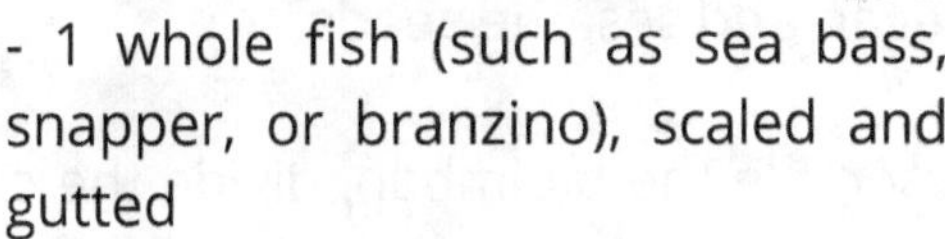

Ingredients:

- 1 whole fish (such as sea bass, snapper, or branzino), scaled and gutted
- 2 tbsp olive oil
- 1 lemon, sliced
- 2 sprigs fresh rosemary
- Salt and pepper to taste

For the Lemon-Herb Butter:
- 4 tbsp unsalted butter, softened
- 2 tbsp chopped fresh parsley
- 1 tbsp chopped fresh dill
- 1 tbsp lemon zest
- 1 tbsp lemon juice
- 1/4 tsp salt

Is the recipe easy to follow?

89. Grilled whole fish

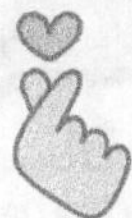

Procedure:

1. Make the lemon-herb butter by mixing together all the ingredients in a small bowl. Set aside.

2. Rinse the whole fish under cold water and pat it dry with paper towels. Use a sharp knife to make a few diagonal slits along the top of the fish.

3. Rub the fish all over with the olive oil and season generously with salt and pepper.

4. Stuff the cavity of the fish with the lemon slices and rosemary sprigs.

5. Preheat a grill or grill pan to medium-high heat. Grease the grates well.

6. Carefully place the whole fish on the hot grill. Cook for 5-7 minutes per side, until the fish flakes easily with a fork.

7. Transfer the grilled fish to a serving platter. Top with dollops of the lemon-herb butter and let it melt over the hot fish.

8. Serve the grilled whole fish immediately, garnished with extra lemon wedges and fresh herbs. Pair with a crisp white wine for a romantic date night meal.

Enjoy this impressive yet easy-to-make grilled whole fish dish!

What is the total cooking time, including prep time?

Prep Time : ______________

Cook Time : ______________

Servings   : ______________

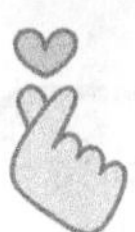

Ingredients:

- 1 cup short-grain brown rice
- 2 cups water
- 1 cup shredded carrots
- 1 cup shredded zucchini
- 1 cup shredded spinach
- 1 cup sliced mushrooms
- 1 cup cubed firm tofu
- 2 tbsp sesame oil
- 2 tbsp soy sauce
- 1 tbsp rice vinegar
- 1 tsp sesame seeds
- 2 eggs
- Gochujang (Korean chili paste), for serving

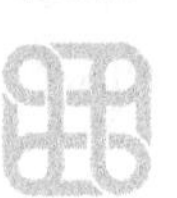
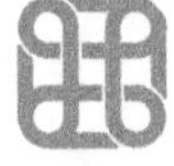
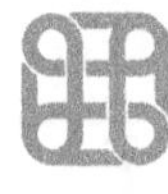
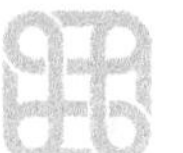

Is the recipe easy to follow?

90. Vegetarian bibimbap

Procedure:

1. Cook the brown rice according to package instructions. Fluff with a fork and set aside.

2. In a large skillet, heat 1 tbsp of the sesame oil over medium-high heat. Add the carrots, zucchini, spinach, and mushrooms. Sauté for 5-7 minutes until vegetables are tender. Season with a pinch of salt and pepper. Transfer to a plate and set aside.

3. In the same skillet, heat the remaining 1 tbsp of sesame oil. Add the cubed tofu and sauté for 3-4 minutes until lightly browned on all sides.

4. In a small bowl, whisk together the soy sauce, rice vinegar, and sesame seeds.

5. To assemble the bibimbap, divide the cooked rice evenly between two large bowls. Top each bowl with the sautéed vegetables, tofu, and a fried egg.

6. Drizzle the soy sauce mixture over the top of each bibimbap bowl.

7. Serve immediately, providing extra gochujang on the side for guests to add as desired.

This colorful and flavorful vegetarian bibimbap makes for a romantic and healthy date night meal. The combination of textures and flavors creates a delicious and visually appealing dish perfect for sharing.

What is the total cooking time, including prep time?

Prep Time : _______________

Cook Time : _______________

Servings   : _______________

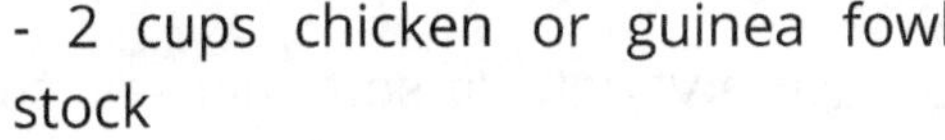

Ingredients:

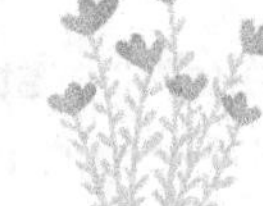

- 1 whole guinea fowl, about 3-4 lbs
- 2 tbsp olive oil
- 2 tsp salt
- 1 tsp black pepper
- 1 lemon, halved
- 4 sprigs fresh thyme
- 2 cloves garlic, peeled and crushed

For the Gravy:
- 2 cups chicken or guinea fowl stock
- 2 tbsp all-purpose flour
- 2 tbsp unsalted butter
- Salt and pepper to taste

Is the recipe easy to follow?

91. Roasted guinea fowl

Procedure:

1. Preheat your oven to 400°F (200°C).

2. Pat the guinea fowl dry with paper towels and place it in a roasting pan. Rub the skin all over with the olive oil and season generously with salt and pepper.

3. Stuff the cavity of the bird with the lemon halves, thyme sprigs, and crushed garlic.

4. Roast the guinea fowl for 60-75 minutes, basting occasionally, until the juices run clear when pierced with a fork and the internal temperature reaches 165°F (75°C).

5. Transfer the roasted guinea fowl to a cutting board and let it rest for 10-15 minutes before carving.

For the Gravy:
1. Pour the pan juices from the roasting pan into a small saucepan. Whisk in the flour and butter until smooth.

2. Gradually whisk in the stock and bring the mixture to a simmer. Cook for 5-7 minutes, stirring frequently, until the gravy has thickened.

3. Season the gravy with salt and pepper to taste.

To Serve:
1. Carve the roasted guinea fowl and arrange the pieces on a serving platter.

2. Serve the guinea fowl warm, with the homemade gravy on the side.

Enjoy this elegant and flavorful roasted guinea fowl dish!

What is the total cooking time, including prep time?

Prep Time : _________________

Cook Time : _________________

Servings : _________________

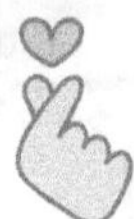

Ingredients:

- 12 fresh figs, halved lengthwise
- 4 oz soft goat cheese, at room temperature
- 2 tbsp honey
- 2 tbsp chopped walnuts
- 1 tbsp chopped fresh thyme
- Pinch of salt

Is the recipe easy to follow?

92. Stuffed figs with goat cheese

Procedure:

1. Preheat your oven to 400°F (200°C).

2. Arrange the fig halves, cut-side up, on a baking sheet lined with parchment paper.

3. In a small bowl, mix together the goat cheese, honey, walnuts, thyme, and a pinch of salt until well combined.

4. Spoon or pipe a small amount of the goat cheese mixture into the center of each fig half, pressing it gently to fill the cavity.

5. Bake the stuffed figs in the preheated oven for 8-10 minutes, or until the cheese is slightly melted and the figs are warm.

6. Remove the stuffed figs from the oven and let them cool for a few minutes.

7. Serve the warm, stuffed figs immediately, either as an appetizer or a light dessert.

Tips:
- Choose fresh, ripe figs for the best flavor and texture.
- You can use a variety of soft cheeses, such as ricotta or mascarpone, in place of the goat cheese.
- Experiment with different nut toppings, such as pecans or almonds, instead of walnuts.
- Drizzle a bit of balsamic glaze over the stuffed figs for an extra touch of sweetness.

These stuffed figs with creamy goat cheese make for a delightful and elegant appetizer or dessert, perfect for entertaining or a romantic date night.

What is the total cooking time, including prep time?

Prep Time : _______________

Cook Time : _______________

Servings   : _______________

Ingredients:

- 8 oz lump crabmeat, picked over for shells
- 1/2 cup panko breadcrumbs
- 2 tbsp mayonnaise
- 1 egg, lightly beaten
- 2 tbsp finely chopped parsley
- 1 tbsp Dijon mustard
- 1 tsp lemon juice
- 1/4 tsp cayenne pepper
- 1/4 tsp salt
- 2 tbsp olive oil

For Serving:
- Lemon wedges
- Tartar sauce or remoulade sauce

Is the recipe easy to follow?

93. Crab cakes

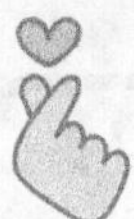

Procedure:

1. In a medium bowl, gently mix together the crabmeat, panko, mayonnaise, egg, parsley, mustard, lemon juice, cayenne, and salt until just combined. Be careful not to break up the crabmeat too much.

2. Divide the crab mixture into 8 equal portions and gently form them into patties, about 3 inches wide and 1/2 inch thick.

3. Heat the olive oil in a large non-stick skillet over medium heat.

4. Working in batches if needed, carefully add the crab cakes to the hot oil and cook for 3-4 minutes per side, until golden brown.

5. Transfer the cooked crab cakes to a paper towel-lined plate.

6. Serve the crab cakes warm, with lemon wedges and tartar or remoulade sauce on the side.

Tips:
- Use high-quality lump crabmeat for the best texture and flavor.
- Gently mix the ingredients to avoid breaking up the crabmeat.
- Chill the crab cake mixture for 30 minutes before forming the patties to help them hold their shape.
- Fry the crab cakes in batches to maintain the oil temperature and ensure even browning.

Enjoy these crispy, flavorful crab cakes as an appetizer or main course!

What is the total cooking time, including prep time?

Prep Time : _______________

Cook Time : _______________

Servings : _______________

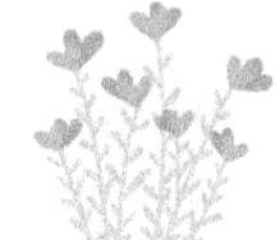

Ingredients:

- 4 medium sweet potatoes
- 2 tbsp olive oil
- 1/2 cup cooked quinoa
- 1/2 cup black beans, drained and rinsed
- 1/4 cup crumbled feta cheese
- 2 tbsp chopped fresh cilantro
- 1 tbsp lime juice
- 1 tsp ground cumin
- Salt and pepper to taste
- Chopped green onions, for garnish

Is the recipe easy to follow?

94. Stuffed sweet potatoes

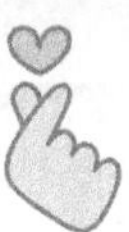

Procedure:

1. Preheat your oven to 400°F. Wash the sweet potatoes and prick them several times with a fork.

2. Place the sweet potatoes directly on the oven rack and bake for 45-60 minutes, until very soft when squeezed. Allow to cool slightly.

3. Slice each sweet potato in half lengthwise. Scoop out the flesh into a medium bowl, leaving a thin layer of sweet potato attached to the skin.

4. In the bowl with the sweet potato flesh, mash it lightly with a fork. Stir in the cooked quinoa, black beans, feta cheese, cilantro, lime juice, and cumin. Season with salt and pepper to taste.

5. Spoon the stuffing mixture back into the sweet potato skins, dividing it evenly among the 8 halves.

6. Place the stuffed sweet potato halves on a baking sheet and return to the oven for 10-15 minutes, until heated through.

7. Carefully transfer the stuffed sweet potatoes to a serving platter. Garnish with chopped green onions.

For a romantic presentation, you can arrange the stuffed sweet potatoes in a circular pattern on a wooden board or platter. The vibrant colors and contrasting textures make this an elegant and visually appealing date night dish.

The combination of the sweet, creamy sweet potato with the savory quinoa, black beans, and tangy feta creates a delicious and satisfying meal. Enjoy these stuffed sweet potatoes together with your partner, perhaps with a side salad and a glass of wine, for a cozy and intimate date night.

What is the total cooking time, including prep time?

Prep Time   : ___________________

Cook Time : ___________________

Servings   : ___________________

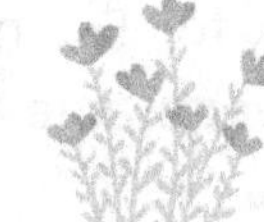

Ingredients:

- 4 boneless, skinless chicken breasts, pounded thin
- 8 thin slices prosciutto
- 8 fresh sage leaves
- 2 tbsp olive oil
- 1/2 cup dry white wine
- 2 tbsp unsalted butter
- 1 tbsp lemon juice
- Salt and pepper to taste

Is the recipe easy to follow?

95. Chicken saltimbocca

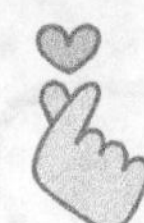

Procedure:

1. Preheat your oven to 400°F (200°C).

2. Season the chicken breasts with salt and pepper on both sides.

3. Place 2 slices of prosciutto on each chicken breast, overlapping slightly. Top each breast with 2 fresh sage leaves.

4. Heat the olive oil in a large, oven-safe skillet over medium-high heat.

5. Carefully add the chicken breasts, prosciutto-side down, and cook for 2-3 minutes until the prosciutto is crispy.

6. Flip the chicken breasts and transfer the skillet to the preheated oven. Roast for 10-12 minutes, or until the chicken is cooked through and reaches an internal temperature of 165°F (75°C).

7. Remove the skillet from the oven and transfer the chicken breasts to a plate. Cover with foil to keep warm.

8. Place the skillet back on the stovetop over medium heat. Add the white wine and use a wooden spoon to scrape up any browned bits from the bottom of the pan.

9. Simmer the wine for 2-3 minutes, then whisk in the butter and lemon juice. Season the sauce with salt and pepper to taste.

10. Serve the chicken saltimbocca immediately, drizzled with the white wine sauce.

Enjoy this elegant and flavorful chicken dish! The prosciutto and sage add a delicious savory element, while the white wine sauce provides a bright, tangy finish.

What is the total cooking time, including prep time?

Prep Time : ___________________

Cook Time : ___________________

Servings   : ___________________

Ingredients:

- 2 medium eggplants, sliced into 1/2-inch rounds
- 2 tbsp olive oil, plus more for brushing
- 1 onion, diced
- 3 cloves garlic, minced
- 1 cup diced zucchini
- 1 cup diced bell pepper
- 1 (15 oz) can diced tomatoes
- 1 tsp dried oregano
- 1/2 tsp ground cinnamon
- Salt and pepper to taste
- 1 cup crumbled feta cheese
- 2 cups béchamel sauce (recipe below)

For the Béchamel Sauce:
- 3 tbsp unsalted butter
- 3 tbsp all-purpose flour
- 2 cups warm milk
- 1/4 tsp ground nutmeg
- Salt and pepper to taste

96. Vegetarian moussaka

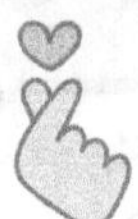

Procedure:

1. Preheat your oven to 375°F (190°C).

2. Brush the eggplant slices with olive oil and arrange them in a single layer on a baking sheet. Roast for 15-20 minutes, flipping halfway, until softened and lightly browned. Set aside.

3. In a large skillet, heat 2 tbsp of olive oil over medium heat. Add the onion and garlic, and sauté for 2-3 minutes until fragrant.

4. Add the zucchini and bell pepper to the skillet. Cook for 5-7 minutes, stirring occasionally, until the vegetables are tender.

5. Stir in the diced tomatoes, oregano, cinnamon, and a pinch of salt and pepper. Simmer for 10 minutes, allowing the flavors to meld.

6. To make the béchamel sauce, melt the butter in a saucepan over medium heat. Whisk in the flour and cook for 2 minutes, stirring constantly. Gradually whisk in the warm milk and cook, stirring frequently, until the sauce thickens, about 5-7 minutes. Season with nutmeg, salt, and pepper.

7. Assemble the moussaka: Arrange a layer of roasted eggplant slices in the bottom of a 9x13-inch baking dish. Top with the vegetable mixture, then sprinkle with the crumbled feta cheese. Pour the béchamel sauce evenly over the top.

8. Bake the moussaka for 30-35 minutes, until the top is golden brown and bubbly.

9. Let the moussaka cool for 10-15 minutes before serving. Enjoy this romantic, vegetarian dish with your partner!

What are the critical points in the recipe (e.g., temperature control, timing)?

What is the total cooking time, including prep time?

Prep Time   : ________________

Cook Time : ________________

Servings   : ________________

Ingredients:

- 1 lb beef tenderloin, trimmed
- 2 tbsp soy sauce
- 1 tbsp rice vinegar
- 1 tbsp sesame oil
- 1 tsp grated ginger
- 1 tsp honey
- 1/4 tsp red pepper flakes (optional)
- 2 tbsp sesame seeds
- 2 green onions, thinly sliced
- Microgreens or sprouts, for garnish

For the Dipping Sauce:
- 2 tbsp soy sauce
- 1 tbsp rice vinegar
- 1 tsp sesame oil
- 1 tsp grated ginger
- 1 tsp honey

Is the recipe easy to follow?

97. Beef tataki

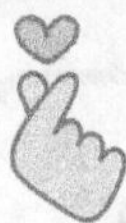

Procedure:

1. In a shallow dish, whisk together the soy sauce, rice vinegar, sesame oil, grated ginger, honey, and red pepper flakes (if using). Add the beef tenderloin and turn to coat evenly. Cover and refrigerate for 30 minutes to 1 hour.

2. In a small bowl, combine the ingredients for the dipping sauce and set aside.

3. Remove the beef from the marinade and pat it dry with paper towels. Heat a large skillet or grill pan over high heat. Sear the beef on all sides until a nice crust forms, about 2-3 minutes per side. The center should still be rare.

4. Transfer the seared beef to a cutting board and let it rest for 5-10 minutes. Slice the beef into thin, diagonal slices.

5. Arrange the sliced beef tataki on a serving platter. Sprinkle with the sesame seeds and green onions.

6. Serve the beef tataki immediately, with the dipping sauce on the side. Garnish with microgreens or sprouts.

7. Encourage your date to dip the beef slices in the sauce and enjoy this elegant, flavorful dish together.

The rare, thinly sliced beef paired with the savory-sweet dipping sauce makes for a romantic and impressive date night meal. Serve with a crisp white wine or sake for a truly special evening.

What are the critical points in the recipe (e.g., temperature control, timing)?

What is the total cooking time, including prep time?

Prep Time : ___________________

Cook Time : ___________________

Servings : ___________________

Ingredients:

- 4 ripe avocados, halved and pitted
- 1 cup cooked quinoa
- 1/2 cup crumbled feta cheese
- 1/4 cup chopped fresh cilantro
- 2 tbsp diced red onion
- 1 tbsp lime juice
- 1 tsp olive oil
- 1/4 tsp ground cumin
- Salt and pepper to taste

For Serving:
- Microgreens or sprouts
- Lime wedges

Is the recipe easy to follow?

🙂 🙁

98. Stuffed avocados

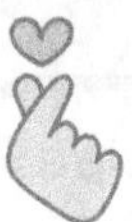

Procedure:

1. In a medium bowl, combine the cooked quinoa, feta cheese, cilantro, red onion, lime juice, olive oil, cumin, and a pinch of salt and pepper. Stir to mix well.

2. Carefully scoop out a small amount of the avocado flesh from each half, leaving a sturdy shell. Chop the scooped-out avocado flesh and add it to the quinoa mixture, gently mixing to incorporate.

3. Spoon the quinoa-avocado mixture evenly into the avocado halves, piling it up slightly.

4. Arrange the stuffed avocado halves on a serving platter. Garnish with microgreens or sprouts and serve with lime wedges.

Tips:
- Choose ripe but firm avocados for the best texture.
- You can use cooked brown rice or couscous instead of quinoa.
- Add diced tomatoes, chopped olives, or sliced jalapeños to the filling for extra flavor.
- Drizzle a bit of balsamic glaze or hot sauce over the top for a flavor boost.

These colorful and nutritious stuffed avocados make for a beautiful and romantic date night appetizer or light main course. The creamy avocado paired with the flavorful quinoa filling creates a delightful contrast in both taste and texture.

What is the total cooking time, including prep time?

Prep Time : _______________

Cook Time : _______________

Servings : _______________

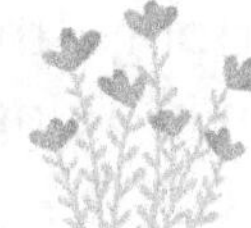

Ingredients:

- 1 lb large shrimp or prawns, peeled and deveined, tails left on
- 2 tbsp olive oil
- 2 tbsp lemon juice
- 2 cloves garlic, minced
- 1 tsp paprika
- 1/2 tsp dried oregano
- 1/4 tsp red pepper flakes (optional)
- Salt and pepper to taste
- Lemon wedges, for serving

For the Garlic Butter Sauce:
- 4 tbsp unsalted butter, softened
- 2 cloves garlic, minced
- 2 tbsp chopped fresh parsley
- 1 tbsp lemon juice
- 1/4 tsp salt

Is the recipe easy to follow?

99. Grilled prawns

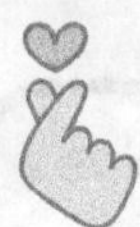

Procedure:

1. In a large bowl, combine the shrimp/prawns, olive oil, lemon juice, garlic, paprika, oregano, red pepper flakes (if using), and a pinch of salt and pepper. Toss to coat the shrimp evenly. Cover and refrigerate for 30 minutes to 1 hour.

2. Make the garlic butter sauce by mixing together the softened butter, minced garlic, parsley, lemon juice, and salt in a small bowl. Set aside.

3. Preheat your grill or grill pan to medium-high heat.

4. Thread the marinated shrimp/prawns onto metal or wooden skewers, leaving a little space between each one.

5. Grill the shrimp skewers for 2-3 minutes per side, or until they are opaque and slightly charred.

6. Transfer the grilled shrimp skewers to a serving platter. Drizzle the garlic butter sauce over the top, allowing it to melt and coat the shrimp.

7. Serve the grilled prawns immediately, with lemon wedges on the side for squeezing over the top.

Tips:
- Use large, fresh shrimp or prawns for the best texture and flavor.
- Marinate the shrimp for at least 30 minutes to infuse them with the garlic and spices.
- Be careful not to overcook the shrimp, as they can become tough and rubbery.
- Serve the grilled prawns with a crisp white wine or a refreshing cocktail for a romantic date night.

Enjoy these flavorful and elegant grilled prawns with your special someone!

What are the critical points in the recipe (e.g., temperature control, timing)?

What is the total cooking time, including prep time?

Prep Time : _______________

Cook Time : _______________

Servings   : _______________

Ingredients:

- 1 jar (16 oz) grape leaves in brine, drained and rinsed
- 1 cup cooked brown rice
- 1/2 cup crumbled feta cheese
- 1/4 cup chopped fresh parsley
- 2 tbsp chopped fresh mint
- 2 tbsp olive oil
- 1 tbsp lemon juice
- 1 clove garlic, minced
- 1/4 tsp ground cinnamon
- Salt and pepper to taste

For the Lemon-Garlic Sauce:
- 1/2 cup plain Greek yogurt
- 2 tbsp lemon juice
- 1 clove garlic, minced
- 1 tbsp chopped fresh dill
- Salt and pepper to taste

Is the recipe easy to follow?

100. Vegetarian stuffed grape leaves

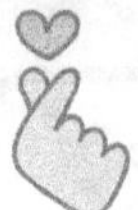

Procedure:

1. In a medium bowl, combine the cooked brown rice, feta cheese, parsley, mint, olive oil, lemon juice, garlic, cinnamon, and a pinch of salt and pepper. Mix well.

2. Lay a grape leaf shiny-side down on a clean work surface. Place about 1-2 tbsp of the rice mixture near the stem end of the leaf. Fold the stem end over the filling, then fold in the sides and tightly roll up the leaf. Repeat with the remaining grape leaves and filling.

3. Arrange the stuffed grape leaves seam-side down in a single layer in a baking dish or platter.

4. In a small bowl, whisk together the ingredients for the lemon-garlic sauce. Season with salt and pepper to taste.

5. Serve the stuffed grape leaves chilled or at room temperature, with the lemon-garlic sauce on the side for dipping.

Tips:
- Use high-quality, brined grape leaves for the best texture and flavor.
- Adjust the amount of filling based on the size of the grape leaves.
- The stuffed grape leaves can be made a day in advance and refrigerated until ready to serve.
- Garnish the platter with fresh herbs, lemon wedges, or edible flowers for a romantic presentation.

These vegetarian stuffed grape leaves make for a delightful and elegant appetizer or light main course for a romantic date night. The combination of the flavorful rice filling and the cool, creamy lemon-garlic sauce is sure to impress your special someone.

What is the total cooking time, including prep time?

Prep Time : _______________

Cook Time : _______________

Servings   : _______________

Ingredients:

- 2 Cornish game hens, about 1-1.5 lbs each
- 2 tbsp olive oil
- 2 tsp dried thyme
- 1 tsp garlic powder
- 1 tsp salt
- 1/2 tsp black pepper
- 1 lemon, halved
- 2 sprigs fresh rosemary

Is the recipe easy to follow?

101. Roasted Cornish game hen

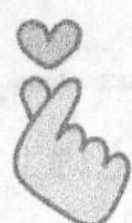

Procedure:

1. Preheat your oven to 400°F (200°C).

2. Pat the Cornish game hens dry with paper towels and place them in a roasting pan or on a rimmed baking sheet.

3. In a small bowl, mix together the olive oil, dried thyme, garlic powder, salt, and black pepper.

4. Rub the seasoning mixture all over the outside of the game hens, making sure to get it into all the nooks and crannies.

5. Place the lemon halves and rosemary sprigs inside the cavities of the game hens.

6. Roast the Cornish game hens in the preheated oven for 45-55 minutes, or until the internal temperature reaches 165°F (75°C) when measured in the thickest part of the thigh.

7. Remove the game hens from the oven and let them rest for 5-10 minutes before serving.

8. To serve, carefully transfer the roasted Cornish game hens to a serving platter. Squeeze the roasted lemon halves over the top, if desired.

Tips:
- For a crispy skin, pat the game hens very dry before seasoning.
- Baste the hens with the pan juices a few times during roasting.
- You can stuff the cavities with additional herbs, garlic, or onion for extra flavor.
- Serve the roasted Cornish game hens with your choice of sides, such as roasted potatoes, sautéed greens, or a fresh salad.

Enjoy this elegant and flavorful roasted Cornish game hen dish for a special occasion or romantic dinner.

What is the total cooking time, including prep time?

Prep Time : _______________

Cook Time : _______________

Servings : _______________

Ingredients:

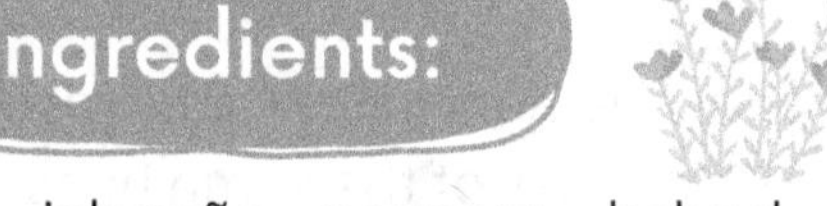

- 12 jalapeño peppers, halved lengthwise and seeded
- 4 oz cream cheese, softened
- 1/2 cup shredded cheddar cheese
- 2 tbsp chopped fresh cilantro
- 1 tbsp lime juice
- 1/4 tsp garlic powder
- Salt and pepper to taste
- 2 tbsp panko breadcrumbs
- 1 tbsp olive oil

For Serving:
- Lime wedges
- Chopped fresh cilantro

Is the recipe easy to follow?

102. Stuffed jalapeño poppers

Procedure:

1. Preheat your oven to 375°F (190°C). Line a baking sheet with parchment paper.

2. In a medium bowl, mix together the cream cheese, cheddar cheese, cilantro, lime juice, garlic powder, and a pinch of salt and pepper until well combined.

3. Carefully spoon or pipe the cheese mixture into the hollowed-out jalapeño halves, filling them evenly.

4. In a small bowl, toss the panko breadcrumbs with the olive oil.

5. Arrange the stuffed jalapeño halves on the prepared baking sheet. Sprinkle the top of each popper with the seasoned panko.

6. Bake the stuffed jalapeño poppers for 15-18 minutes, or until the filling is heated through and the panko is golden brown.

7. Remove the poppers from the oven and let them cool for a few minutes.

8. Arrange the warm, stuffed jalapeño poppers on a serving platter. Garnish with additional chopped cilantro and serve with lime wedges.

Tips:
- Wear gloves when handling the jalapeños to avoid skin irritation.
- For a milder flavor, use a combination of jalapeños and bell peppers.
- Experiment with different cheese fillings, such as cream cheese and goat cheese or cheddar and Parmesan.
- Serve the stuffed jalapeño poppers with a refreshing cocktail or a crisp white wine for a romantic date night.

What is the total cooking time, including prep time?

Prep Time : ________________

Cook Time : ________________

Servings   : ________________

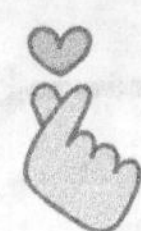

Ingredients:

- 2 live lobsters (about 1 lb each)
- 4 tbsp unsalted butter
- 1 onion, diced
- 2 carrots, peeled and diced
- 2 celery stalks, diced
- 3 garlic cloves, minced
- 1/4 cup dry white wine
- 4 cups seafood or chicken stock
- 1 cup heavy cream
- 2 tbsp tomato paste
- 1 tsp paprika
- 1/4 tsp cayenne pepper
- Salt and pepper to taste
- Chopped chives, for garnish

Is the recipe easy to follow?

103. Lobster bisque

Procedure:

1. Bring a large pot of salted water to a boil. Add the live lobsters and cook for 8-10 minutes, until they turn bright red. Remove the lobsters from the water and let them cool slightly.

2. Once the lobsters are cool enough to handle, twist off the tails and claws. Remove the meat from the shells and set aside. Reserve the shells.

3. In a large pot or Dutch oven, melt the butter over medium heat. Add the onion, carrots, celery, and garlic. Sauté for 5-7 minutes, until the vegetables are softened.

4. Add the reserved lobster shells to the pot and pour in the white wine. Simmer for 2-3 minutes, scraping up any browned bits from the bottom of the pot.

5. Pour in the seafood or chicken stock and bring the mixture to a boil. Reduce the heat and let the bisque simmer for 30 minutes, allowing the flavors to meld.

6. Remove the lobster shells from the pot. Use an immersion blender to puree the soup until smooth.

7. Stir in the heavy cream, tomato paste, paprika, and cayenne. Season with salt and pepper to taste.

8. Gently fold in the cooked lobster meat and let the bisque simmer for an additional 5-10 minutes, until heated through.

9. Ladle the lobster bisque into bowls and garnish with chopped chives.

10. Serve the romantic lobster bisque warm, with crusty bread or crackers on the side.

What are the critical points in the recipe (e.g., temperature control, timing)?

What is the total cooking time, including prep time?

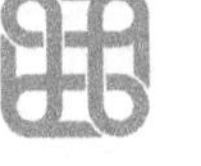 Prep Time : _______________

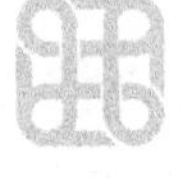 Cook Time : _______________

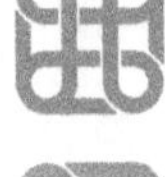 Servings : _______________

Ingredients:

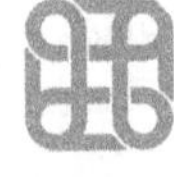

- 1 medium butternut squash, halved lengthwise and seeded
- 2 tbsp olive oil, plus more for drizzling
- 1 cup cooked wild rice or quinoa
- 1/2 cup crumbled feta cheese
- 1/4 cup chopped walnuts
- 2 tbsp dried cranberries
- 2 tbsp chopped fresh parsley
- 1 tsp dried thyme
- Salt and pepper to taste
- Balsamic glaze, for drizzling (optional)

Is the recipe easy to follow?

104. Stuffed butternut squash

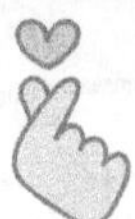

Procedure:

1. Preheat your oven to 400°F (200°C).

2. Place the butternut squash halves cut-side up on a baking sheet. Drizzle with olive oil and season with salt and pepper.

3. Roast the squash in the preheated oven for 40-50 minutes, or until fork-tender.

4. In a medium bowl, combine the cooked wild rice or quinoa, feta cheese, walnuts, dried cranberries, parsley, and thyme. Season with salt and pepper.

5. Once the squash is cooked, remove it from the oven and let it cool slightly. Reduce the oven temperature to 375°F (190°C).

6. Scoop out the flesh from the squash halves, leaving a 1/2-inch border around the edges to create a "boat." Mash the scooped-out flesh and add it to the rice/quinoa mixture. Stir to combine.

7. Spoon the stuffing mixture back into the squash halves, piling it up slightly.

8. Return the stuffed squash halves to the baking sheet and bake for an additional 15-20 minutes, until the filling is heated through and the edges are lightly browned.

9. Remove the stuffed squash from the oven and let it cool for a few minutes.

10. Drizzle the stuffed squash with a bit of balsamic glaze, if desired. Serve warm, garnished with extra parsley or thyme.

What is the total cooking time, including prep time?

Prep Time : ________________

Cook Time : ________________

Servings   : ________________

Ingredients:

- 4 veal cutlets, pounded thin (about 1/4 inch thick)
- 1 cup all-purpose flour
- 2 eggs, beaten
- 1 cup panko breadcrumbs
- 1/2 cup grated Parmesan cheese
- 1 tsp dried parsley
- 1/2 tsp garlic powder
- Salt and pepper to taste
- Vegetable oil for frying
- Lemon wedges, for serving

For the Arugula Salad:
- 4 cups baby arugula
- 1 tbsp olive oil
- 1 tbsp lemon juice
- Salt and pepper to taste

Is the recipe easy to follow?

105. Veal Milanese

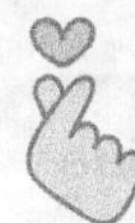

Procedure:

1. Set up a breading station with three shallow dishes: one with the flour, one with the beaten eggs, and one with the panko breadcrumbs mixed with the Parmesan, parsley, garlic powder, salt, and pepper.

2. Dredge the veal cutlets in the flour, dip them in the egg, and then coat them evenly with the seasoned breadcrumb mixture, pressing gently to adhere.

3. In a large skillet, heat about 1/4 inch of vegetable oil over medium-high heat.

4. Working in batches, fry the breaded veal cutlets for 2-3 minutes per side, until golden brown and crispy. Transfer the fried veal to a paper towel-lined plate.

5. In a medium bowl, toss the baby arugula with the olive oil, lemon juice, and a pinch of salt and pepper.

6. To serve, place the veal Milanese on plates and top with the arugula salad. Garnish with lemon wedges.

Tips:
- Pound the veal cutlets thin to ensure even cooking and a crispy texture.
- Use high-quality veal for the best flavor and tenderness.
- Fry the veal in batches to maintain the oil temperature and achieve the perfect crispiness.
- Serve the veal Milanese immediately for the best texture.
- Pair the dish with a crisp white wine or a light, refreshing cocktail for a romantic date night.

This classic Italian dish of crispy, golden-brown veal Milanese paired with a fresh arugula salad makes for an elegant and impressive romantic dinner. Enjoy this flavorful and indulgent meal with your special someone.

What is the total cooking time, including prep time?

Prep Time : _______________

Cook Time : _______________

Servings   : _______________

Ingredients:

- 2 tbsp coconut oil
- 1 onion, diced
- 3 cloves garlic, minced
- 1 tbsp grated fresh ginger
- 2 tsp garam masala
- 1 tsp ground cumin
- 1 tsp ground coriander
- 1/2 tsp ground turmeric
- 1/4 tsp cayenne pepper (or to taste)
- 1 (15 oz) can diced tomatoes
- 1 (13.5 oz) can coconut milk
- 1 cup vegetable broth
- 1 medium sweet potato, peeled and cubed
- 1 cup cauliflower florets
- 1 cup frozen peas
- 1 (15 oz) can chickpeas, drained and rinsed
- Salt and pepper to taste
- Chopped cilantro for garnish
- Cooked basmati rice, for serving

106. Vegetarian curry

Procedure:

1. In a large pot or Dutch oven, heat the coconut oil over medium heat. Add the onion and sauté for 5 minutes until translucent.

2. Add the garlic and ginger and cook for 1 minute, until fragrant.

3. Stir in the garam masala, cumin, coriander, turmeric, and cayenne. Cook for 2 minutes to toast the spices.

4. Pour in the diced tomatoes, coconut milk, and vegetable broth. Bring the mixture to a simmer.

5. Add the cubed sweet potato, cauliflower florets, frozen peas, and chickpeas. Season with salt and pepper.

6. Reduce the heat to medium-low and let the curry simmer for 20-25 minutes, or until the vegetables are tender.

7. Taste and adjust seasoning as needed.

8. Serve the vegetarian curry over steamed basmati rice, garnished with chopped cilantro.

Tips:
- Use a variety of vegetables like bell peppers, spinach, or eggplant to customize the curry.
- For a creamier curry, use full-fat coconut milk.
- Adjust the amount of cayenne pepper to control the spice level.
- Serve with naan bread, chutney, or raita for a complete Indian-inspired meal.

This flavorful vegetarian curry is a comforting and satisfying dish that's perfect for a romantic date night or a cozy dinner at home.

What is the total cooking time, including prep time?

Prep Time : _______________

Cook Time : _______________

Servings   : _______________

Ingredients:

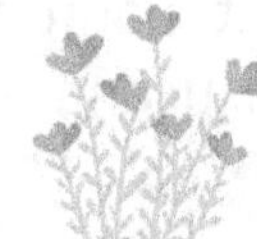

- 8 oz beef tenderloin, trimmed of fat and sinew
- 2 tbsp olive oil
- 1 tbsp lemon juice
- 1 tsp Dijon mustard
- 1 tsp capers, drained and chopped
- 1 tsp chopped fresh parsley
- Salt and pepper to taste
- Arugula or mixed greens
- Shaved Parmesan cheese
- Lemon wedges, for serving

Is the recipe easy to follow?

107. Beef carpaccio

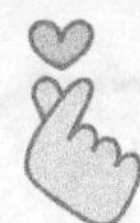

Procedure:

1. Place the beef tenderloin in the freezer for 30-60 minutes to firm up slightly, making it easier to slice.

2. In a small bowl, whisk together the olive oil, lemon juice, Dijon mustard, capers, and parsley. Season with a pinch of salt and pepper.

3. Remove the beef from the freezer and, using a very sharp knife, slice it into paper-thin slices. Arrange the slices in a single layer on a large plate or platter.

4. Drizzle the lemon-caper dressing evenly over the beef carpaccio.

5. Top the carpaccio with a bed of arugula or mixed greens. Shave Parmesan cheese over the top.

6. Cover the platter with plastic wrap and refrigerate for 30 minutes to 1 hour, allowing the flavors to meld.

7. Remove the carpaccio from the fridge about 10 minutes before serving to allow it to come closer to room temperature.

8. Serve the beef carpaccio immediately, garnished with additional lemon wedges.

Tips:
- Use the freshest, highest-quality beef tenderloin for the best flavor and texture.
- Slice the beef as thinly as possible, almost translucent, for the classic carpaccio presentation.
- Adjust the amount of lemon juice and capers to your taste preferences.
- Garnish with other toppings like shaved truffles, toasted pine nuts, or a drizzle of truffle oil for added elegance.

What is the total cooking time, including prep time?

Prep Time : ______________

Cook Time : ______________

Servings : ______________

Ingredients:

- 4 large bell peppers (any color), halved lengthwise and seeded
- 1 cup cooked brown rice
- 1 lb ground turkey or lean ground beef
- 1 small onion, finely chopped
- 2 cloves garlic, minced
- 1 (14.5 oz) can diced tomatoes
- 1/2 cup shredded mozzarella cheese
- 2 tbsp chopped fresh basil
- 1 tsp dried oregano
- Salt and pepper to taste

For Serving:
- Grated Parmesan cheese
- Chopped fresh parsley

Is the recipe easy to follow?

108. Stuffed bell peppers

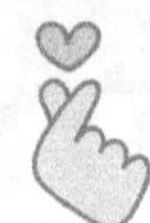

Procedure:

1. Preheat your oven to 375°F (190°C).

2. Arrange the bell pepper halves in a baking dish or on a rimmed baking sheet, cut-side up.

3. In a large skillet, cook the ground turkey or beef over medium heat, breaking it up with a wooden spoon, until browned and cooked through, about 5-7 minutes. Drain any excess fat.

4. Add the chopped onion and garlic to the skillet. Sauté for 2-3 minutes until the onion is translucent.

5. Stir in the cooked brown rice, diced tomatoes, 1/4 cup of the mozzarella cheese, basil, oregano, and a pinch of salt and pepper. Mix well.

6. Spoon the filling evenly into the bell pepper halves, packing it down gently.

7. Top the stuffed peppers with the remaining 1/4 cup of mozzarella cheese.

8. Bake the stuffed peppers in the preheated oven for 25-30 minutes, or until the peppers are tender and the cheese is melted and bubbly.

9. Remove the stuffed peppers from the oven and let them cool for a few minutes.

10. Serve the stuffed bell peppers warm, garnished with grated Parmesan cheese and chopped fresh parsley.

Tips:
- Choose bell peppers that are similar in size for even cooking.
- Substitute the ground meat with cooked lentils or crumbled tofu for a vegetarian version.
- Add sautéed mushrooms, spinach, or diced zucchini to the filling for extra flavor and nutrition.

What is the total cooking time, including prep time?

Prep Time : _______________

Cook Time : _______________

Servings : _______________

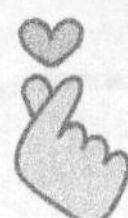

Ingredients:

- 4 (6 oz) sea bass fillets, skin-on
- 2 tbsp olive oil
- 2 tbsp lemon juice
- 2 tsp minced garlic
- 1 tsp dried oregano
- 1/2 tsp salt
- 1/4 tsp black pepper
- Lemon wedges, for serving

For the Lemon-Herb Butter:
- 4 tbsp unsalted butter, softened
- 2 tbsp chopped fresh parsley
- 1 tbsp chopped fresh dill
- 1 tbsp lemon zest
- 1 tbsp lemon juice
- 1/4 tsp salt

Is the recipe easy to follow?

109. Grilled sea bass

Procedure:

1. Make the lemon-herb butter by mixing together all the ingredients in a small bowl. Set aside.

2. In a shallow baking dish, combine the olive oil, lemon juice, garlic, oregano, salt, and pepper. Add the sea bass fillets and turn to coat them evenly in the marinade. Cover and refrigerate for 30 minutes to 1 hour.

3. Preheat your grill or grill pan to medium-high heat.

4. Remove the sea bass fillets from the marinade and place them skin-side down on the hot grill. Cook for 4-5 minutes per side, or until the fish flakes easily with a fork.

5. Transfer the grilled sea bass to a serving platter. Top each fillet with a dollop of the lemon-herb butter, allowing it to melt over the hot fish.

6. Serve the grilled sea bass immediately, garnished with lemon wedges.

Tips:
- Choose fresh, high-quality sea bass fillets for the best flavor and texture.
- Marinate the fish for at least 30 minutes to infuse it with the lemon and herb flavors.
- Be careful not to overcook the sea bass, as it can become dry and tough.
- Serve the grilled sea bass with a side of roasted vegetables, a fresh salad, or steamed rice for a complete romantic meal.
- Pair the dish with a crisp white wine or a light, refreshing cocktail for a truly special date night.

This elegant and flavorful grilled sea bass with lemon-herb butter makes for a romantic and impressive date night dinner. Enjoy the delicate, flaky fish with your special someone.

What is the total cooking time, including prep time?

Prep Time : _______________

Cook Time : _______________

Servings   : _______________

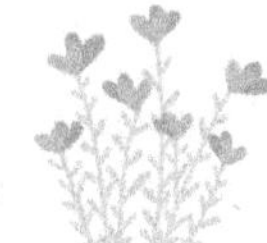

Ingredients:

- 12 lasagna noodles
- 1 (15 oz) container ricotta cheese
- 1 cup shredded mozzarella cheese, divided
- 1/2 cup grated Parmesan cheese
- 1 egg
- 2 cups chopped spinach
- 1 cup diced mushrooms
- 2 cloves garlic, minced
- 1 tsp dried basil
- 1/2 tsp dried oregano
- Salt and pepper to taste
- 2 cups marinara sauce

Is the recipe easy to follow?

110. Vegetarian lasagna rolls

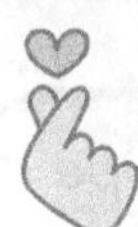

Procedure:

1. Preheat your oven to 375°F (190°C).

2. Bring a large pot of salted water to a boil. Cook the lasagna noodles according to package instructions until al dente. Drain and rinse with cold water.

3. In a medium bowl, mix together the ricotta cheese, 1/2 cup of the mozzarella, Parmesan, egg, spinach, mushrooms, garlic, basil, oregano, and a pinch of salt and pepper.

4. Spread about 2-3 tablespoons of the ricotta mixture onto each cooked lasagna noodle, then roll them up tightly.

5. Spread 1 cup of the marinara sauce in the bottom of a 9x13-inch baking dish. Arrange the lasagna rolls seam-side down in the dish.

6. Pour the remaining 1 cup of marinara sauce over the top of the lasagna rolls, making sure to cover them completely.

7. Sprinkle the remaining 1/2 cup of mozzarella cheese over the top.

8. Bake the lasagna rolls in the preheated oven for 25-30 minutes, or until the cheese is melted and bubbly.

9. Remove the lasagna rolls from the oven and let them cool for 5 minutes.

10. Serve the vegetarian lasagna rolls warm, garnished with additional fresh basil or parsley, if desired.

Tips:
- Use no-boil lasagna noodles to save time and effort.
- Experiment with different vegetable fillings, such as roasted red peppers, zucchini, or eggplant.

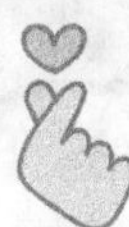

Procedure:

1. Preheat your oven to 400°F (200°C).

2. Rub the quail all over with the olive oil and season generously with salt and pepper.

3. Place the quail on a baking sheet or in a roasting pan, making sure they are not touching each other.

4. Roast the quail in the preheated oven for 20-25 minutes, or until the juices run clear when pierced with a fork.

5. Remove the quail from the oven and let them rest for 5 minutes.

6. Serve the roasted quail warm, with the lemon wedges on the side for squeezing over the top.

Enjoy your delicious roasted quail!

What is the total cooking time, including prep time?

Prep Time : _________________

Cook Time : _________________

Servings : _________________

Ingredients:

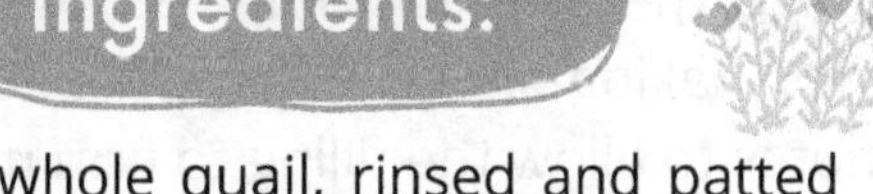

- 4 whole quail, rinsed and patted dry
- 2 tbsp olive oil
- 1 tsp salt
- 1/2 tsp black pepper
- 1 lemon, cut into wedges (for serving)

Is the recipe easy to follow?

111. Roasted quail

What are the critical points in the recipe (e.g., temperature control, timing)?

What is the total cooking time, including prep time?

Prep Time : _______________

Cook Time : _______________

Servings   : _______________

Ingredients:

- 20-24 cherry tomatoes
- 4 oz cream cheese, softened
- 2 tbsp grated Parmesan cheese
- 1 tbsp chopped fresh basil
- 1 tsp garlic powder
- 1/4 tsp salt
- 1/8 tsp black pepper

Is the recipe easy to follow?

112. Stuffed cherry tomatoes

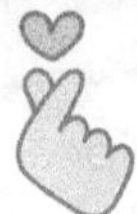

Procedure:

1. Wash the cherry tomatoes and slice off the top 1/4 inch of each tomato. Carefully scoop out the seeds and pulp from the center, leaving a small hollow in each tomato.

2. In a small bowl, mix together the cream cheese, Parmesan, basil, garlic powder, salt, and pepper until well combined.

3. Using a small spoon or piping bag, fill each hollowed-out tomato with the cream cheese mixture, mounding it slightly on top.

4. Arrange the stuffed tomatoes on a serving platter or baking sheet. Refrigerate for at least 30 minutes to allow the filling to firm up.

5. Serve the stuffed cherry tomatoes chilled or at room temperature. They make a great appetizer or side dish.

Variations:
- Try using different herbs like chives, dill, or parsley instead of basil.
- Add a small piece of cooked bacon or crumbled feta cheese on top.
- For a spicy kick, mix in a pinch of cayenne pepper or crushed red pepper flakes.

Enjoy your delicious stuffed cherry tomatoes!

What is the total cooking time, including prep time?

Prep Time : _______________

Cook Time : _______________

Servings   : _______________

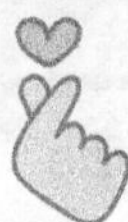

Ingredients:

- 2 tbsp olive oil
- 1 onion, diced
- 3 cloves garlic, minced
- 1 fennel bulb, diced
- 1 cup dry white wine
- 1 (28 oz) can diced tomatoes
- 2 cups seafood or vegetable broth
- 1 tsp dried oregano
- 1 tsp dried basil
- 1/2 tsp red pepper flakes (optional)
- 1 lb mussels, scrubbed and debearded
- 1 lb large shrimp, peeled and deveined
- 1 lb white fish fillets (such as cod, halibut or sea bass), cut into 1-inch pieces
- 1 lb lump crabmeat
- Salt and pepper to taste
- Chopped parsley for garnish

Is the recipe easy to follow?

113. Seafood cioppino

Procedure:

1. In a large pot or Dutch oven, heat the olive oil over medium heat. Add the onion, garlic and fennel. Cook for 5-7 minutes until softened.

2. Pour in the white wine and let it simmer for 2-3 minutes to cook off the alcohol.

3. Add the diced tomatoes, broth, oregano, basil and red pepper flakes (if using). Bring to a simmer.

4. Add the mussels, shrimp, fish and crabmeat. Cover and cook for 8-10 minutes, until the mussels have opened and the seafood is cooked through.

5. Season with salt and pepper to taste.

6. Ladle the cioppino into bowls and garnish with chopped parsley. Serve with crusty bread for dipping.

Enjoy this hearty and flavorful seafood stew! The combination of mussels, shrimp, white fish and crab makes it a real seafood lover's delight.

What is the total cooking time, including prep time?

Prep Time : _______________

Cook Time : _______________

Servings   : _______________

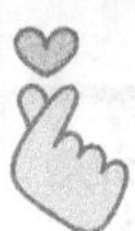

Ingredients:

- 2 acorn squash, halved and seeded
- 2 tbsp olive oil
- Salt and pepper to taste
- 1 lb Italian sausage, casings removed
- 1 onion, diced
- 3 cloves garlic, minced
- 1 cup cooked wild rice
- 1/2 cup dried cranberries
- 1/2 cup toasted pecans, chopped
- 1/4 cup grated Parmesan cheese
- 2 tbsp chopped fresh parsley

Is the recipe easy to follow?

114. Stuffed acorn squash

Procedure:

1. Preheat oven to 400°F. Place the acorn squash halves cut-side up on a baking sheet. Drizzle with olive oil and season with salt and pepper. Roast for 30-40 minutes, until tender when pierced with a fork.

2. In a skillet over medium heat, cook the Italian sausage, breaking it up as it cooks, until browned and cooked through, about 8-10 minutes. Drain excess fat.

3. Add the onion and garlic to the skillet and cook for 3-4 minutes until softened.

4. In a bowl, mix together the cooked sausage mixture, wild rice, cranberries, pecans, Parmesan and parsley.

5. Scoop the stuffing mixture evenly into the roasted acorn squash halves.

6. Return the stuffed squash to the oven and bake for an additional 15-20 minutes, until the squash is very tender and the stuffing is hot.

7. Serve the stuffed acorn squash warm, garnished with extra parsley if desired.

The sweet roasted squash pairs beautifully with the savory sausage, rice and nut stuffing. This makes a wonderful fall or winter side dish or even a main course.

What is the total cooking time, including prep time?

Prep Time : _______________

Cook Time : _______________

Servings   : _______________

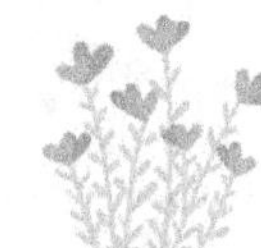

Ingredients:

- 4 boneless, skinless chicken breasts
- 4 tbsp unsalted butter, softened
- 2 cloves garlic, minced
- 2 tbsp chopped fresh parsley
- 1/4 tsp salt
- 1/8 tsp black pepper
- 1 cup all-purpose flour
- 2 eggs, beaten
- 1 cup panko breadcrumbs

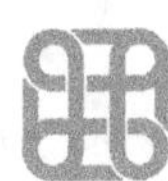
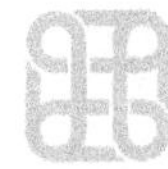
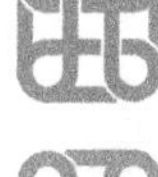
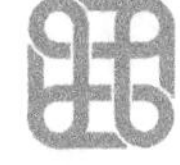
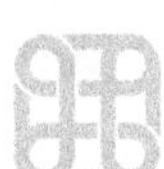

Is the recipe easy to follow?

115. Chicken Kiev

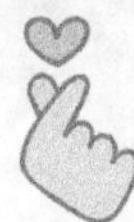

Procedure:

1. Pound the chicken breasts between two sheets of plastic wrap or parchment paper until they are about 1/4 inch thick. Set aside.

2. In a small bowl, mix together the softened butter, garlic, parsley, salt and pepper until well combined.

3. Spoon about 1 tbsp of the garlic-herb butter onto the center of each chicken breast. Fold the sides of the chicken over the butter to enclose it completely, then secure with toothpicks.

4. Set up a breading station with the flour, beaten eggs and panko breadcrumbs in separate shallow dishes.

5. Dredge the stuffed chicken breasts first in the flour, shaking off any excess. Then dip them in the beaten egg, allowing any excess to drip off. Finally, coat them thoroughly in the panko breadcrumbs.

6. Place the breaded chicken breasts on a baking sheet or plate and refrigerate for at least 30 minutes to help the coating set.

7. Preheat oven to 400°F.

8. Bake the chicken kiev for 25-30 minutes, until the chicken is cooked through and the coating is golden brown.

9. Remove the toothpicks and serve the chicken kiev immediately, allowing the garlic-herb butter to ooze out when cut into.

Enjoy this classic, elegant chicken dish! The crispy breading and melted butter filling make it a true comfort food favorite.